Patient Alcohol Abuse

A Guide for Health Care Professionals

Author

FAITH S. SCHAEFER, BS

Consulting Editor

MILTON E. BURGLASS, MD

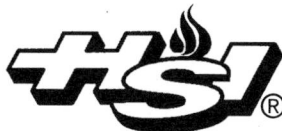

Health Studies Institute, Inc.

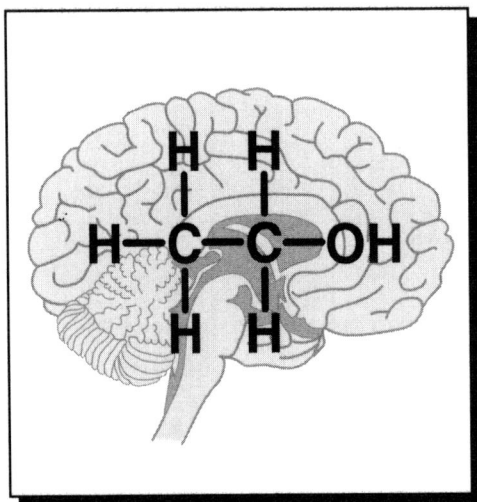

Cover: The structural formula for alcohol is superimposed on a drawing of the brain. Alcohol affects all parts of the body, but its gargantuan cost to society is mainly caused by its effect on the brain.

Patient Alcohol Abuse

A Guide for Health Care Professionals

Milton Earl Burglass, MD, MPH, MDiv, MS, CAS, CMRO, FAAFP, FASAM, is a Fellow of the American Society of Addiction Medicine and is a member of the clinical and research faculties at the Zinberg Center for Addiction Studies, Harvard Medical School. He serves as treatment provider and consultant to the judicial, corrections, alcohol and drug treatment, mental health, DUI, and professional regulatory agencies in Massachusetts, Rhode Island, and Florida. He is also on the faculties of the University of Miami and the University of Massachusetts. He has been a psychiatrist for the adult and juvenile court clinic systems in Massachusetts, and is qualified as an expert on psychiatry and substance abuse by the criminal and civil courts in 24 states, throughout the federal court system, and in Canada.

Dr. Burglass has been on the faculties of the Department of Psychiatry, Harvard Medical School at the Cambridge Hospital; Boston University; Tufts University; the University of Miami Department of Religion; and Harvard Divinity School. At present, he serves as special consultant to the Vatican State, on public health programming for alcohol and drug treatment services in Central and South America. He serves the governments of Spain, Argentina, Uruguay, and Brazil in the same capacity.

An internationally recognized expert on substance abuse, Dr. Burglass is specifically concerned with methadone treatment, impaired professionals, and forensic addiction medicine. He frequently contributes articles on addictions, neuropsychiatry, theology, information science, and law to professional journals.

Faith Sousa Schaefer holds a BS in Communications from Florida International University, and did her graduate work in adult education. From 1971 to 1994, she worked on the International Oceanographic Foundation's magazine, *Sea Frontiers,* first as Associate Editor, then as Senior Editor. She joined Health Studies Institute's staff in 1994, as a researcher, writer, and editor. Ms. Schaefer has published many articles, especially on marine science, and is the author of *Family Violence: Responding to Signs of Abuse in Your Patients.*

A special thank you to **Joan Schulman**, MA, our senior staff editor, for her many contributions and guidance in developing this text.

Published by Health Studies Institute, Inc.
P.O. Box 163200
Miami, FL 33116-3200

ISBN 1-879772-09-4

9 781879 772090

Contents

Algorithms

Figures

Tables of Information

Directions

How to Get the Most Out of This Course

Become completely familiar with the material in each chapter before going on to the next. First, preview by skimming the chapter; then read it. Study the tables, algorithms, illustrations, and appendices, and use the Definitions, Abbreviations, and Acronyms, and the Index in the back of the book to aid your understanding. Finally, quiz yourself, using the review questions between chapters to evaluate your mastery of the material. Go at your own pace.

The Post-Test

Please use a No. 2 pencil to fill out the Scantron answer form for the post-test. There are 50 questions; a passing grade requires 40 correct answers. Keep a copy of your answers for your own records. If you fail the post-test, you may retake it for a $5.00 service charge. Each question has only one correct answer; there are no trick questions and no deliberate fogginess. If you see a way to improve our questions, please note your suggestions on the certificate request form.

Certification

The purchase of a course entitles only one person, the named purchaser, to receive continuing education credit. If we don't have your name registered, we cannot send your certificate. We keep records for licensure and certification; please notify us if your name or address changes.

If you need a replacement certificate, we are glad to provide one. The replacement fee of $5 includes mailing and handling. Your state licensing board may request your certificate of completion, or a copy of it, so file it carefully.

Mailing Instructions

1. Make sure your name and the course title appear correctly on the post-test answer form.
2. Complete the certificate request form.
3. Mail both of these forms to: Health Studies Institute
   P.O. Box 163200
   Miami, FL 33116-3200

We will mail your certificate promptly upon receipt of the answer form and certificate request. If you don't receive your certificate, please notify us: 1-800-700-3454. Thank you for continuing your professional education with us.

Health Studies Institute, Inc.

Objectives

At the end of this course, you will take a written test which will measure your ability to identify:

1. Categories of alcohol misuse
2. Milestones in society's handling of alcohol misuse
3. Current alcohol-related problems
4. Population groups identified as misusers of alcoholic beverages
5. Theories on why people misuse alcohol
6. Processes involved in alcohol metabolism
7. Effects of rising blood alcohol concentration
8. Diagnostic criteria for alcohol abuse and dependence
9. Clinical procedures identifying patients who misuse alcohol
10. Clinical intervention techniques
11. Confidentiality laws
12. Alcohol's effect on the nervous system
13. Characteristics of alcohol-induced neurologic and psychologic disorders
14. Characteristics of alcohol-related physiologic disorders
15. Medications which interact adversely with alcohol
16. Treatments of alcohol withdrawal syndrome
17. Chemical, supportive, and behavioral techniques for preventing relapse

Introduction

In the course of your life, you have almost certainly encountered at least one person who misused alcohol (i.e., ethanol or ethyl alcohol). Perhaps it was a loud-mouthed guy guzzling beer next to you at the football game, a homeless girl drinking cheap wine under an expressway overpass, or a group of teenagers passing around a bottle of bourbon in a cruising car. It could even have been your socially proper spouse or parent who sat quietly before the TV each night, sipping shot after shot of whiskey, before staggering to the bedroom.

> Only when one considers the potential of alcohol misuse is its societal impact apparent.

Sadly, society in general views such actions as simply "the way things are." Only when one considers the potential of alcohol misuse is its societal impact apparent. Did the intoxicated football fan beat up his wife when he got home? Did the homeless girl infect a stranger with human immunodeficiency virus (HIV) while having sex to get money for her next bottle? Did the teenagers, while driving home, run a red light and kill someone in another vehicle? Will your spouse or parent die prematurely because alcohol misuse has impaired the functioning of various body organs?

> Alcohol, a very simple molecule, has a complex and tenacious grip on many Americans.

Alcohol, a very simple molecule (see cover), has a complex and tenacious grip on many Americans; approximately 25% of adults either have alcohol-related problems or have drinking patterns putting them at risk for developing such problems.[1] Each year in the United States, alcohol misuse is related to an estimated 100,000 deaths (many of them traffic fatalities) and some $86 billion in costs.[2] Intoxicated persons often suffer trauma, engage in unsafe sex, rob or attack strangers, or commit acts of family violence. Signs of alcohol use are found in the offender, victim, or both in about half of all homicides and serious assaults. Thousands of children exposed to alcohol prenatally suffer congenital defects, growth retardation, and learning disabilities—all of them preventable.

Many persons who misuse alcohol do not seek the health care they need. However, between 20% and 30% of all persons who do seek any primary health care have alcohol-related disorders, ranging from the physiologic to the neurologic and psychologic.[3] These same patients often consult a wide range of clinicians, including dental workers, nurses, therapists, and counselors, who provide specialized care.

> All health care workers, except those dealing with very young children, have patients who misuse alcohol.

Therefore, <u>all</u> health care workers, except those dealing with very young children, have patients who misuse alcohol, and, no matter what your clinical practice, it is your responsibility to identify these patients and take the appropriate actions.

This course offers suggestions on how you can:

- Avoid administering or prescribing any medication whose interaction with alcohol in patients' blood could have grave consequences
- Identify patients' alcohol misuse, demonstrate concern, and refer the patients to addiction specialists (which you can and should do, according to experts on addiction medicine)

> Current medical policy encourages clinical intervention during the initial stage of alcohol misuse.

Current medical policy encourages clinical intervention during the initial stage of alcohol misuse. Even <u>brief</u> clinician-patient discussions can affect patients' drinking habits, because they realize that someone is genuinely concerned about their health.[1] In other words, only clinical interventions which are attempted have any chance of helping patients.

This course covers patients' alcohol misuse and the related harmful effects; in ascending order of seriousness, the misuse categories are:

1. <u>Hazardous drinking</u>—drinkers do <u>not yet</u> have alcohol-related problems, but occasionally increase their risk of harm when they drink, then engage in certain activities (e.g., driving, swimming, unprotected sex).

2. <u>Mild alcohol problems</u>—drinkers' lives are negatively affected (e.g., injuries, arrests, family disputes); however, the problems are not as serious as those which accompany alcohol abuse.

3. <u>Alcohol abuse</u>—despite persistent or recurrent interpersonal or social problems (e.g., arrests for drunk driving, physical fights, serious marital difficulties), drinkers continue to drink to excess.

> **Note:** *This course uses the term <u>alcohol abuse</u> only when discussing this specific category of alcohol misuse; <u>alcohol misuse</u> refers to any excessive drinking (e.g., binge, chronic, or heavy drinking) or clearly destructive drinking (e.g., any sneaking or even sipping of alcohol by persons who are pregnant or recovering from alcohol abuse or dependence). Definitions of drinking patterns (binge, chronic, moderate, heavy, social, and very heavy) vary greatly in medical literature; brief explanations of each drinking pattern appear in "Definitions, Abbreviations, and Acronyms" in this book.*

4. Alcohol <u>dependence</u> (often called <u>alcoholism</u> in the medical literature)—drinkers have developed clinically significant impairment or distress, manifesting particular symptoms, e.g.:

   - Tolerance—needing markedly greater amounts or more frequent consumption of alcohol to achieve intoxication
   - Withdrawal—experiencing a characteristic physiologic syndrome when chronic drinking is stopped or interrupted
   - Impaired control—failing to manage alcohol use, despite the desire to cut down on drinking
   - Preoccupation with drinking—spending a great deal of time on activities related to drinking
   - Drinking despite problems—continuing to drink though aware of persistent physiologic or mental disorders, caused or exacerbated by the alcohol.[2,4]

An estimated 7.4% of Americans meet the American Psychiatric Association's diagnostic criteria for alcohol abuse or alcohol dependence.[5] (*See Chapter 5.*) Although the health care community cannot agree on whether alcohol dependence is a disease or a habit, this disorder gradually destroys the physical and mental health of its victims.

> Clinicians may see or hear something that arouses their suspicions, then ask a nonjudgmental, open-ended question inviting conversation.

This course first summarizes the history of the use and regulation of beverage alcohol, reviewing demographic trends and discussing some of the many reasons people drink alcohol. This material provides an understanding of how alcohol misuse became the grave societal problem it is today. The course then explores what clinicians, <u>regardless of their specialties</u>, can do to prevent or reduce patient alcohol misuse. For example, while treating patients, clinicians may see or hear something that arouses their suspicions, then ask a nonjudgmental, open-ended question inviting conversation: "Do you enjoy having a drink or two occasionally?" How to inject such questions tactfully into conversations, as well as how to employ many other techniques to treat patients who misuse alcohol, are the heart of the course. Health care workers, in accordance with their clinical practices and training, can:

- <u>Identify</u> patients who misuse alcohol, at the earliest possible stages, using screening techniques and diagnostic assessments
- <u>Intervene</u> by educating, encouraging, and motivating patients to overcome their denial of alcohol misuse and obtain addiction treatment
- <u>Recognize</u> signs and symptoms of mental and physiologic disorders
- <u>Refer</u> patients appropriately, then cooperate with the addiction specialists by motivating patients during subsequent visits to the referring clinicians.

Whether patients have been drinking recently or chronically also affects the treatment clinicians offer. Clinicians <u>must</u> avoid giving intoxicated patients any medications which interact adversely with alcohol, could create a medical emergency, or could prevent the patient from driving home safely. The following scenarios illustrate how the information this course provides can prove invaluable to any clinician.

> *A patient arrives late for his 3 p.m. appointment, exclaiming that his business lunch took a lot longer than he expected. The receptionist asks him to take a seat, then turns to you and says: "Did you get a whiff of that guy?"*

Be on the lookout for: signs of intoxication. A patient who is mildly or moderately intoxicated may smell of alcohol, talk loudly and profusely, be unsteady when standing, and lack coordination.
If you find confirming evidence, be aware that: The patient has alcohol in his blood (blood alcohol concentration, BAC), which can interact adversely with other drugs used during clinical treatment. Do you know which medications can trigger an exaggerated or overdose-like response in an intoxicated patient? (*See Table 19, Chapter 11.*)

> *A scrawny patient with yellowed skin arrives for an emergency molar extraction. She says she feels like throwing up and has abdominal pain. Her history form indicates that she "takes a drink now and then."*

Be on the lookout for: alcoholic hepatitis or cirrhosis. Patients with these serious disorders may be jaundiced and have lost weight; they may complain of nausea, vomiting, and dull abdominal pain.
If you find confirming evidence, be aware that: the patient is a chronic drinker whose liver function has been compromised by alcohol. Do you know why local anesthetics such as lidocaine and mepivacaine

could be toxic to such patients? Do you know why chronic drinkers heal more slowly, which could create problems after tooth extractions? (*See Oral Disorders, Chapter 10.*)

> At 8 a.m. on a Monday, two frantic students rush into the college clinic, carrying a friend who has been drinking all night; he now has trouble breathing and is afraid that he's having a heart attack.

Be on the lookout for: cardiac arrhythmias. A patient who has been binge drinking can develop these symptoms.
If you find confirming evidence, be aware that: a high incidence of sudden death has been associated with binge drinking. (*See Cardiovascular Disease, Chapter 10.*) Do you know what societal problems are associated with binge drinking, and how widespread it is? (*See Student Binge Drinking, Chapter 2.*)

> Upon entering the examination room, you observe that a patient's hands are shaking as she holds a cup of water, and drops of sweat are streaming down her face. Her chart shows that her pulse rate and temperature are elevated.

Be on the lookout for: alcoholic withdrawal syndrome. Most patients undergoing the syndrome respond to supportive measures; however, some require medications for seizures, hallucinations, and delirium tremens.
If you find confirming evidence, be aware that: the patient may have suddenly quit her daily, very heavy drinking so she could sober up for the visit. Do you know that certain medications you might administer or prescribe can cause shock or coma if the patient's BAC is >0.15 g/dL? Do you know what precautions to take if she is seizure-prone? (*See Withdrawal and Medical Detoxification, Chapter 12.*)

> A well-groomed patient arrives for an employer-required physical examination. He is articulate, well-coordinated, and mentally alert, but, while taking his blood pressure, you see that he has facial rosacea and rhinophyma.

Be on the lookout for: tolerance to alcohol. Chronic drinking can accelerate the metabolism of alcohol, reducing its intoxicating effects and behavioral signs. Clinicians may have to rely on physiologic signs such as facial rosacea, nystagmus, or Dupuytren's contracture. (*See Table 14, Chapter 6.*)

If you find confirming evidence, be aware that: the patient could have a high BAC and not exhibit obvious signs of intoxication. Do you know how to ask tactfully about alcohol use while taking a patient history? (*See Patient History, Chapter 6.*) Do you know which molecules in blood are tested for signs of recent or chronic drinking? (*See Biological State Markers, Chapter 6.*)

> *Concerned about a patient's unsuccessful attempts to quit drinking, you diplomatically suggest that he attend an Alcoholics Anonymous (A.A.) meeting.*

Be on the lookout for: unfounded objections to attending A.A. meetings. A patient might say: "Then everybody will know I'm a drunk," or "I don't need all that religion."

If you find confirming evidence, be aware that: the patient doesn't understand the Twelve Steps and Traditions of A.A. Can you respond effectively and informatively to the patient's objections? (*See Twelve-Step Programs, Chapter 13.*)

Ultimately, the patient must make the decision to seek help, but you can assist by providing information and encouragement. Detecting alcohol misuse is one of your professional obligations; ensuring that the patients who have such problems can make informed decisions about the path they will take is also your professional duty. This course will help you perform both tasks.

Chapter 1   Historical and Societal Perspectives

Alcohol is produced by fermentation; this occurs naturally when airborne yeasts act on substances containing sugar (e.g., a mash of grapes or honey), left exposed in a warm atmosphere. Prehistoric people probably discovered alcohol and its intoxicating effects by accident. However, they soon learned to produce wines and beers, which assumed a major role in social and religious ceremonies. This chapter provides a brief history of alcohol use and its effects on society, from ancient times to the present.

Legends and Myths

> The epic of Gilgamesh associates wine with sacrificial blood, a symbolism preserved by many religions today.

On stone tablets and papyrus scrolls, early literate societies recorded legends about alcoholic beverages. In the Babylonian epic of Gilgamesh, the bodies of benevolent gods, killed in battle against the powers of evil, are consumed by Earth to produce grape vines. This legend associates wine with sacrificial blood, a symbolism preserved by many religions today.[6]

In the Homeric Hymns (circa 800 B.C.), according to the Greek god Dionysus during his travels to India and Thrace, the "vine" was a blend of good in moderation and evil in excess. However, the Romans replaced Dionysus with the god Bacchus, who approved of excessive wine consumption. In the Ovidian *Metamorphoses* (1st century A.D.), Bacchus is delighted when Midas and Silenus try to outdrink each other for 10 days.[6]

Earliest Records

Records of actual alcohol consumption date from 4000 B.C. Mesopotamian clay tablets contain recipes for using wine as a solvent in medicines. Egyptian papyrus scrolls indicate that beer was an important commercial product. Early Hebrew records reveal that this society used several types of wine, each for a distinct ceremonial purpose.[6]

Alcoholic Beverage Development

In the Middle Ages, wine-making improved greatly when Crusaders brought the sirah grape from Persia to France. In the 8th century A.D., Arabian alchemist Geber (Jabir ibn Hayyan) perfected a wine distillation process. By the 12th century, distillation was used to make whiskey in Scotland and Ireland, countries with climates not suitable for growing grapes. In the 17th century, the Dutch chemist Sylvius produced gin, flavoring the alcohol with juniper to disguise its taste. The English government encouraged use of Sylvius's profitable distillation procedure, a decision which proved disastrous for England. By 1742, English gin production reached 20 million gallons per year, and alcoholism was widespread among the lower classes, as illustrated in William Hogarth's images of "Gin Lane" and described in Charles Dickens's novels.[6]

> By 1742, English gin production reached 20 million gallons per year, and alcoholism was widespread among the lower classes.

In the 1600s, Dutch settlers in New York established a gin distillery, although, in the American colonies, rum made from molasses ("rumbullion") was a more profitable commodity. New England distillers set up a "triangle trade": the molasses, imported from the West Indies, was distilled into rum, which was then shipped to Africa and traded for slaves, who were then brought to the West Indies to be traded for molasses. This industry came to a halt when Congress outlawed slave trading in 1808. As a result, other American distillers, previously operating in isolated areas, found a widespread and profitable market for bourbon, rye, and corn whiskey.[6]

Laws and Temperance Movements

An increase in drinking accompanied the production and distillation improvements, and governments of the time, like those of earlier eras, recognized the need for control. Table 1 shows some of the regulations, dating from 1700 B.C.—1933 A.D., aimed at restricting the consumption of alcohol. Temperance movements predate Christianity; the Egyptian *Wisdom of Ani* and the Chinese *Canon of History* (circa 650 B.C.) caution against excessive drinking. The Old Testament contains many similar warnings, which undoubtedly contributed to the traditional antipathy toward inebriation in the Jewish culture.[6] Centuries ago, Buddhism banned consumption of alcohol, a practice continued today by devout followers of this religion. (*See Table 1.*)

Table 1. Regulation of Alcohol Consumption
Notable Laws, 1700 B.C.—1933 A.D.

Countries	Regulations
Babylonia	Circa 1700 B.C., the Code of Hammurabi restricted sale and consumption of alcohol; violators of certain public drinking house laws were executed.
China	Circa 1700 B.C., drunkards were executed to demonstrate the government's disapproval of alcohol consumption.
Greece	Circa 800 B.C., Greek regulations mandated fines for drunkards, specified dilutions of wine with water, and provided wine inspectors; drinking of undiluted wine was considered uncivilized.
India	In the 5th century B.C., Buddhist sects banned alcohol consumption.
Rome	By 186 B.C., excessive drinking had overwhelmed conversation at intellectual symposiums, so the Roman Senate banned them; in 81 A.D., Emperor Domitian ordered that half the country's vineyards be destroyed (no new vines were planted until 276 A.D.).
Switzerland	In 1226, Switzerland passed tavern closing time laws.
England	In 1285, the government enacted laws setting pub closing times. By 1742, gin production had reached 20 million gallons per year, and excessive consumption of gin was causing grave societal problems; the government levied high taxes on alcoholic beverages and began to engineer a shift of national drinking preferences from distilled beverages to ale and beer.
Scotland	In 1436, Scotland passed tavern closing time laws.
United States	In 1919, Congress passed the 18th amendment to the Constitution, which prohibited the manufacture and sale of "intoxicating liquors," starting 1 year from its ratification; the amendment was enforced by the Volstead Act. In 1933, Congress passed the 21st amendment, repealing Prohibition.

The first formal temperance society, the Order of St. Christopher, was founded in Germany in 1517 A.D. Soon afterward, societies stressing more moderate consumption were established in many other countries in which distilled liquors were popular.[6]

> Colonial societies considered the problem to be the person who used the alcohol, not the alcohol itself.

In the United States, major changes in the perception of alcohol misuse occurred between colonial times and the beginning of the temperance movements in the 1800s. Colonial societies considered the problem to be the <u>person</u> who used the alcohol, not the alcohol itself. Habitual drunkenness, viewed as a character weakness and a sin against God and the church, was punished by confinement in stocks.[6]

During the 19th century, as America metamorphosed from an agrarian to an industrial society, poverty and crime grew. These social ills were seen as connected to the use of alcoholic beverages, and many local groups were formed to fight "demon rum" by advocating moderate ("temperate") drinking. In the 1850s, organizations such as the American Temperance Society, the Women's Christian Temperance

Union, and the Anti-Saloon League fought against <u>any</u> use of alcoholic beverages.[7] By 1912, a number of states had enacted prohibition laws, paving the way for passage of the 18th amendment to the Constitution, in 1919, establishing national Prohibition.[6]

Transition to Modern Times

In 1933, the 21st amendment to the Constitution ended Prohibition in the United States. During its early years, Prohibition succeeded in some ways: fewer deaths from liver cirrhosis were reported, and arrests for public drunkenness were greatly reduced.[8] Ultimately, however, Prohibition failed because many Americans considered it an intolerable infringement of personal freedom; they made their own alcoholic beverages or frequented illegal speakeasies, supplied with smuggled or "bootleg" liquor by violent criminal elements. However, despite its failures, Prohibition did stimulate scientific study of alcohol misuse, previously considered a moral failing.

> Prohibition failed because many Americans considered it an intolerable infringement of personal freedom.

As early as the late 1700s, Benjamin Rush of Philadelphia had identified alcoholism as a disease, characterized by loss of control over drinking behavior and curable only by abstinence. In the 1900s, E. M. Jellinek further refined this disease concept, hoping to increase much-needed medical services for alcoholics. He used the term "alcoholism" only when persons had:

1. Impaired ability to stop drinking
2. Developed tolerance to alcohol
3. Experienced signs and symptoms of alcohol withdrawal syndrome.[9]

Even today, these symptoms are among those included in the American Psychiatric Association's and World Health Organization's diagnostic criteria for alcohol dependence. (*See Table 11, Chapter 5.*)

Changing Attitudes

In 1935, Alcoholics Anonymous (A.A.) was founded. This fellowship demonstrated that alcoholics <u>could</u> recover, which helped to stimulate national policy debate on alcohol-related problems. Table 2 shows milestones on the road to understanding, starting in 1935.[2,7,10]

A major milestone was the creation of the National Institute on Alcohol Abuse and Alcoholism (NIAAA) by Congress in 1970. Since then, thanks to NIAAA support, researchers have made significant strides in understanding the causes, prevention, and treatment of alcohol dependence and its consequences. NIAAA-supported research also led, in 1981, to the Surgeon General's issuance of a health advisory on the risk of drinking during pregnancy.[11]

Table 2. Alcohol-related Milestones	
Dates	**People and Organizations**
June 11, 1935	Alcoholics Anonymous (A.A.) was founded by stockbroker William Griffith Wilson and Dr. Robert H. Smith.
Mid-1930s	The Research Council on Problems of Alcohol was created at Yale University; in 1940, the Council began publication of the *Quarterly Journal of Studies on Alcohol.*
1944	The National Committee for Education on Alcohol was founded by A.A. member Marty Mann and Yale University researchers; the Committee was later renamed the National Council on Alcoholism.
1950s	The World Health Organization and the American Medical Association began to address health care aspects of alcohol dependence and discrimination against alcoholics in health care settings; soon afterward, the American Psychiatric Association and the American Public Health Association began similar work.
1965	The National Center for the Prevention and Control of Alcohol Problems, part of the National Institute of Mental Health (NIMH), was established, with a limited budget.
July 30, 1969	The Senate Special Subcommittee on Alcoholism and Narcotics held its first hearing on alcohol misuse and related problems.
1970	On May 14, Senator Harold Hughes introduced S. 3835, a bill intended to provide a comprehensive federal program for prevention and treatment of alcoholism; on December 15, a modified version of the bill passed the House of Representatives as Public Law 91-616; on December 31, President Nixon signed the bill, which created the National Institute on Alcohol Abuse and Alcoholism (NIAAA) as a branch of NIMH.
1974	Passage of Public Law 93-282 created the Alcohol, Drug Abuse, and Mental Health Administration, comprising three institutes: NIAAA, NIMH, and the National Institute on Drug Abuse (NIDA).
Early 1980s	The organizations called Mothers Against Drunk Driving (MADD) and Students Against Driving Drunk (SADD) were formed. Subsequently, legislators passed the Federal Uniform Drinking Age Act of 1984, specifying that federal highway funds would be withheld from any state which did not set 21 as the minimum legal drinking age for purchase or public possession of any type of alcoholic beverage.
1988	Congress passed Public Law 100-960 requiring that, starting in 1989, alcoholic beverage containers carry a label: **GOVERNMENT WARNING: (1) ACCORDING TO THE SURGEON GENERAL, WOMEN SHOULD NOT DRINK ALCOHOLIC BEVERAGES DURING PREGNANCY BECAUSE OF THE RISK OF BIRTH DEFECTS. (2) CONSUMPTION OF ALCOHOLIC BEVERAGES IMPAIRS YOUR ABILITY TO DRIVE A CAR OR OPERATE MACHINERY, AND MAY CAUSE HEALTH PROBLEMS.**

Current Societal Problems

Research has repeatedly documented high rates of alcohol involvement in a wide range of serious and/or fatal injury events, including motor vehicle crashes, noncommercial aviation crashes, drownings, bicycle accidents, domestic violence, suicides, and homicides.[2]

Motor Vehicle Crashes

In a study of 201 automobile drivers admitted to Tennessee emergency rooms for trauma, Kirby et al.[12] found that, of the victims, 37% had a positive blood alcohol concentration (BAC)—and 37% of the latter tested positive for other drugs as well. Based on these findings, the American Medical Association (AMA) recommends that all trauma victims (including drivers) of legal drinking age (≥21) be screened for drugs. Therefore, when health care workers note recent alcohol or other drug use by any trauma victims, they should, in addition to treating the acute medical emergency, provide referrals for substance abuse evaluation.[13]

> NHTSA estimates that, since 1979, alcohol has been involved in almost 45% of deaths caused by automobile accidents.

U.S. alcohol-related motor vehicle crashes cost an estimated $46 billion annually, when emergency services, medical treatment, property damage, lost productivity, travel delay, and legal services are considered. Since 1979, an average of 45,000 people per year have died in automobile accidents in the United States, and the National Highway Traffic Safety Administration (NHTSA) estimates that alcohol has been involved in almost 45% of these deaths.

From 1979 to 1992, there was a 30% decrease in the number of male drivers involved in U.S. alcohol-related fatal crashes, but a 4% increase in the number of female drivers so involved.[5,14] During 1992, 37.4% of total U.S. traffic fatalities were alcohol-related; during 1994, the percentage increased to 40.8%. NHTSA considers a police-reported fatal crash to be alcohol-related if either the driver or a nonoccupant (e.g., pedestrian, cyclist) has a BAC of ≥0.01 g/dL; the driver may or may not have been killed in the crash. (In the literature, BAC is expressed in various ways, as shown in Table 3.)

Table 3. BAC Equivalents			
Percent	Grams/deciliter	Milligrams/deciliter	Milligrams/100 milliliters
0.10%	0.10 g/dL	100 mg/dL	100 mg%

Most states define intoxication while operating a motor vehicle or boat as having a BAC of ≥0.10 g/dL; however, the following states have already lowered the standard to ≥0.08 g/dL: California, Florida, Kansas, Maine, New Hampshire, New Mexico, North Carolina, Oregon, Utah, Vermont, and Virginia. For drivers <21 years of age, about 70% of states have set special BAC limits ranging from 0 to 0.002 g/dL (0.002 g/dL allows for alcohol in medications or sacramental wine).

Fig. 1 graphs the proportion, by age group, of total 1995 traffic fatalities reported by NHTSA. The data show that, in the 25-34 age group, 59% (4,654) of the fatalities were alcohol related (BAC ≥0.01 g/dL) compared with 41% (3,253) which were non-alcohol related (BAC none). Of the 4,654 alcohol-related fatalities, 83% had a BAC of ≥0.10 g/dL, which equals the legal intoxication level in most states.

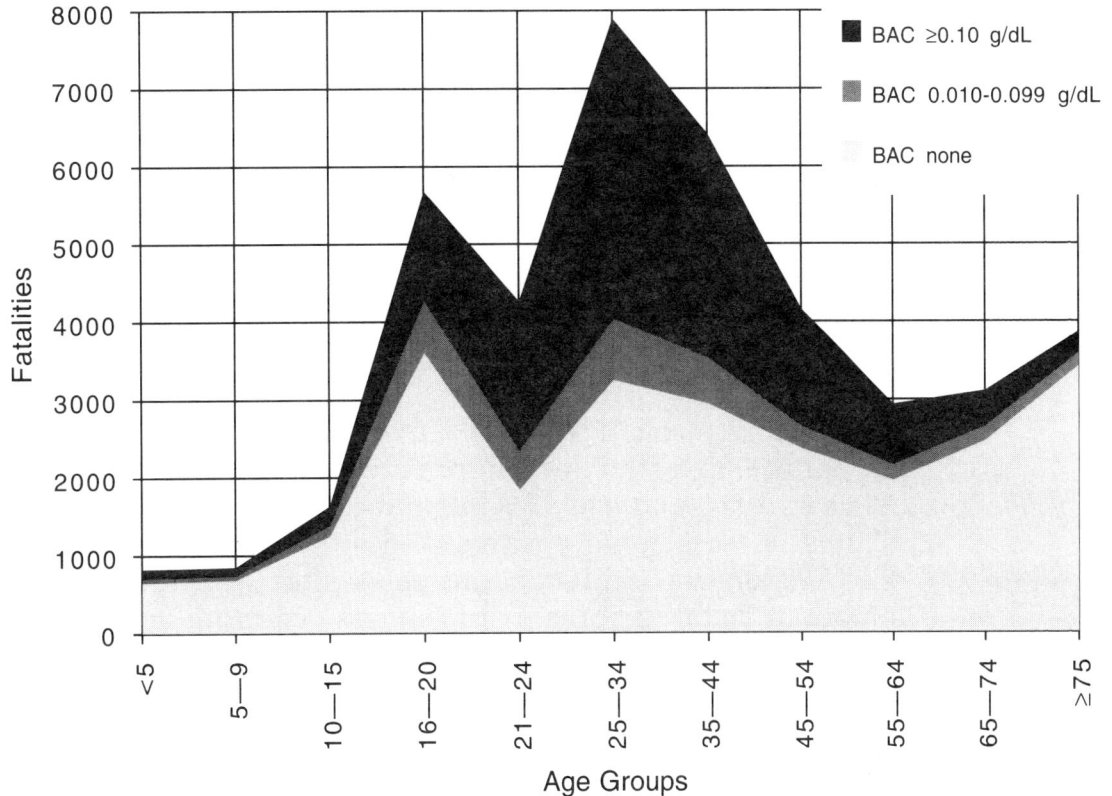

Fig. 1. Total 1995 Traffic Fatalities, Alcohol and Non-Alcohol Related

Violence

Alcohol is associated with a substantial number of violent acts, during which intoxicated persons inflict bodily harm, e.g., on family members in the privacy of their homes, or on friends and strangers in public. Based on examination of interview data collected from 1,887 felons convicted of homicides, Wieczorek et al.[15] found that more than half of the offenders were under the influence of alcohol, illegal drugs, or both, at the time of the crime. Welte and Abel[16] report that alcohol use was a likely factor in homicides emerging spontaneously from personal disputes; victims typically included:

1. People killed by stabbing, or
2. People killed in bars and restaurants, or
3. People killed on Saturday and Sunday nights, or
4. Males killed by females.[2]

Other Problem Areas

Typical estimates of noncommercial aviation crashes in which pilots died and alcohol was involved range from 10% to 30%. Oosterveld[17] reported that increased gravity forces associated with flight can produce positional alcohol nystagmus (PAN) up to 48 hours after a pilot consumes alcohol; PAN may contribute to some aviation crashes involving spatial disorientation. In a study of the effects of alcohol on the ability of pilots to communicate by radio, Morrow et al.[18] found that BACs as low as 0.04 g/dL significantly impaired pilot performance. The researchers also found evidence of "hangover effects"; pilots' radio communication was adversely affected 8 hours after they had registered a BAC of 0.10 g/dL.

An estimated 47% to 65% of adult drownings are associated with alcohol use. In a study of California coroners' reports on 234 drownings between 1974 and 1985, Wintemute et al.[19] found that 41% of the victims tested alcohol positive, and, of these, 30% had BACs of ≥0.10 g/dL. Emerging evidence indicates that alcohol may also be an important factor in spinal cord injuries occurring during shallow-water diving.[2]

Chapter Summary

1. The earliest records of actual alcohol consumption, Mesopotamian clay tablets dating from 4000 B.C., give recipes for using wine as a solvent in medicines.

2. In colonial America, rum was made from molasses and traded for slaves; the profitable industry came to a halt when Congress outlawed slave trading in 1808.

3. The first formal temperance society, the Order of St. Christopher, was founded in Germany in 1517; American societies, formed in the 1800s, initially advocated moderate ("temperate") drinking, but later rejected <u>any</u> use of alcoholic beverages.

4. American temperance societies helped to influence Congress to pass, in 1919, the 18th amendment to the Constitution, prohibiting the manufacture and sale of "intoxicating liquors." In 1933, however, Congress repealed Prohibition by passing the 21st amendment.

5. Although Prohibition failed to prevent all manufacture and sale of alcoholic beverages, it did stimulate the study of alcohol misuse in America.

6. Alcoholics Anonymous (A.A.) was founded in 1935 by stockbroker William Griffith Wilson and Dr. Robert H. Smith.

7. In 1988, Congress passed Public Law 100-960, requiring alcoholic beverage containers to carry warnings against drinking during pregnancy and before driving a car or operating machinery.

8. During 1995, the greatest number of traffic fatalities associated with BACs of $\geq$0.01 g/dL involved persons aged 25-34; of these 4,654 persons, 83% had a BAC of $\geq$0.10 g/dL.

9. A recent study of 1,887 felons convicted of homicides showed that, at the time of the crime, more than half of the offenders were under the influence of alcohol, illegal drugs, or both.

10. A study of 234 drownings in California between 1974 and 1985 showed that 30% of the victims had BACs of $\geq$0.10 g/dL.

Chapter 2   Alcohol Use Epidemiology

The primary goal of alcohol epidemiology is to identify and explain the factors which underlie alcohol use and misuse, and how these factors affect various populations. Researchers achieve this goal via:

1. Surveillance—tracking per capita alcohol consumption and related factors (e.g., increases and decreases in alcohol-related traffic fatalities or use of treatment services for alcohol dependence)
2. Survey research—studies which correlate each respondent's drinking patterns with other personal data (e.g., family history of alcohol misuse).[5]

Such data can then be used to develop effective prevention, counseling, and/or treatment strategies for patients who misuse alcohol or may do so.

Alcohol-Use Surveillance

Fig. 2 shows, for 1935 through 1992, the average number of gallons of <u>pure</u> (or absolute) alcohol consumed per person age ≥14 in the United States.

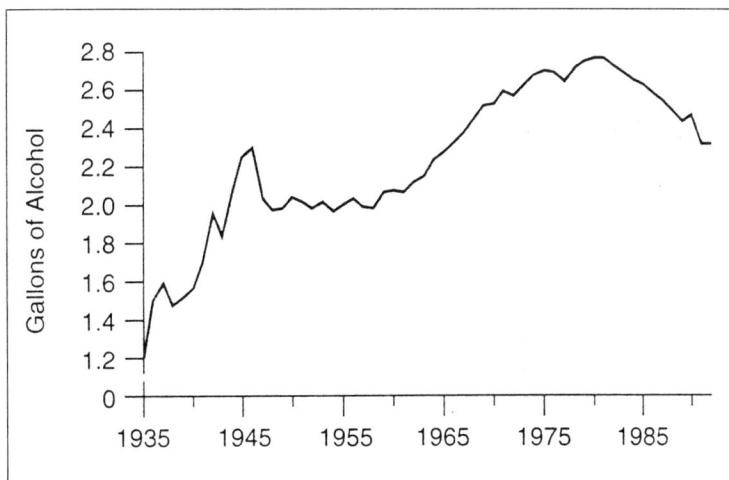

Fig. 2. Per Capita Alcohol Consumption, U.S., 1935-1992: the average number of gallons of pure alcohol, for all types of alcoholic beverages

The figure was calculated by multiplying total gallons of each beverage type by an <u>average</u> "percent alcohol" (beers, 4.5%; wines, 12.9%; liquors, 41.4%), then summing all types.[20,21] (*See Table 8, Chapter 4, for calculation on a per-drink basis.*) Fig. 2 data, calculated using beverage sales data from the 50 states and the District of Columbia, do not include estimates of alcohol produced at home or illegally, or untaxed alcohol brought into the United States by tourists.[5]

| After repeal of Prohibition in 1933, per capita alcohol consumption increased, reaching about 2.3 gallons following World War II. |

As Fig. 2 shows, after repeal of Prohibition in 1933, per capita alcohol consumption increased (with some fluctuation), reaching about 2.3 gallons following World War II. After a modest decrease in the 1950s, it increased again, peaking in 1980-1981 at just below 2.8 gallons. For the remainder of the 1980s, per capita consumption showed a 12% decrease, the only sustained decrease since Prohibition; by 1991, it had decreased to 2.31 gallons, the lowest level since 1965.[5]

The 1992 National Longitudinal Alcohol Epidemiologic Survey (NLAES) showed an 8% decrease, since 1988, in the number of current drinkers (i.e., persons who had consumed at least 12 drinks in the prior 12 months). The survey also showed that, in general, the number of current drinkers decreased with advancing age, increased with higher income and education, was lower in the South than in other regions, and was lower in rural than in urban areas.[5]

| Approximately 25% of the total U.S. population aged ≥18 used alcohol ≥51 days during 1995. |

Table 4 shows results of the 1995 National Household Survey on Drug Abuse, sponsored by the Substance Abuse and Mental Health Services Administration (SAMHSA). The data indicate that approximately 25% of the total U.S. population aged ≥18 used alcohol ≥51 days during 1995. However, these figures do not include military personnel on active duty, transient populations (e.g., homeless people not residing in shelters), and residents of institutional group quarters (e.g., jails and hospitals).[22]

Gender and Age Factors

Studies of alcohol use, in the United States and other countries, have consistently found that men drink more than women and experience more adverse consequences.[2] According to the data in Table 4, during 1995, the highest percentages of males and females using alcohol ≥51 days occurred in the 26-34 age group. This correlates closely with the fact that members of the 25-34 age group were involved in the greatest number of alcohol-related traffic fatalities. (*See Fig. 1,*

Table 4. Alcohol Use in the United States, 1995

Categories of Drinkers		Alcohol Used at Least Once During 1995		Alcohol Used ≥51 Days During 1995	
		No. of Users (estimate, in thousands)	% of U.S. Population (in category)	No. of Users (estimate, in thousands)	% of U.S. Population (in category)
Gender and Age	**Males**				
	12-17	4,015	35.3	680	6.0
	18-25	11,069	80.4	4,506	32.7
	26-34	14,221	80.8	6,703	38.1
	≥35	41,745	71.1	20,502	34.9
	Females				
	12-17	3,777	34.8	388	3.6
	18-25	10,216	72.7	2,145	15.3
	26-34	13,482	73.3	3,117	17.0
	≥35	39,790	59.6	10,597	15.9
Race or Ethnicity (by gender)	**Whites**				
	Males	55,827	72.5	26,223	34.0
	Females	54,116	65.4	13,967	16.9
	African Americans				
	Males	6,216	58.5	2,862	26.9
	Females	6,532	50.0	1,396	10.7
	Hispanics				
	Males	6,913	70.4	2,613	26.6
	Females	4,518	45.6	540	5.4

Chapter 1.) In the ≥35 age group, the percentage of males drinking ≥51 days during 1995 is slightly more than twice that of females.[22]

Population studies have not documented an increase in heavy drinking by females in general; however, increases have been found within certain subgroups of women:

1. Mercer and Khavari[23] found that, among college students they surveyed, females consumed as much beer or wine at one sitting as males, or even more, particularly if the quantities were corrected for gender differences in body water and fatty tissue.[24] (*See Blood Alcohol Concentration, Chapter 4*.)

2. LaRosa[25] found that women working in nontraditional, male-dominated occupations (e.g., high-ranking female executives) were more likely than other employed women of comparable age and education to drink excessively.[26]

Student Binge Drinking

Drinking ≥5 drinks consecutively, on one occasion, is called binge drinking. In the University of Michigan's Monitoring the Future Study for 1991, 30% of American high school seniors surveyed reported episodes of binge drinking during the prior 2 weeks. Thirty-eight percent of male high school seniors reported such episodes, compared with 21% of female seniors.[27]

Binge drinking is widespread on many American college campuses; however, it varies with the type of college, the geographical location, and the student population's ethnicity and gender. In 1994, 40% of college students surveyed reported binge drinking at least once during the prior 2 weeks. A comparison of college students and nonstudents aged 18 to 21 revealed more binge drinking among the students. Table 5 shows the distribution of college student binge drinking.[28]

Table 5. College Student Binge Drinking	
Distribution by:	**Estimated Percentages of Student Populations**
Gender	• Male: 52% • Female: 31% (percentage probably is low because, considering physiologic gender differences, a more equivalent binge-drinking criterion for women is four drinks, rather than five, per occasion)
Race or Ethnicity	• In one multicampus survey: 43.8% of Whites; 40.6% of Native Americans; 31.3% of Hispanics; 22.7% of Asians; 22.5% of African Americans

Research shows that, as a consequence of binge drinking, college students may:

1. Experience sexual assaults—about 50% of female sexual assault victims at one university had been binge drinking.
2. Act aggressively—67% of male aggressors at one university had been binge drinking at the time of the assault or incident of victimization.
3. Drive after drinking—reported by 60% of college men and almost 50% of college women who binge drink on at least three occasions during a 2-week period.[28]

Persons involved in binge drinking may also suffer a higher than average number of injuries, miss classes, disturb other students, and damage property. They may engage in unplanned sexual activity, abandoning safe sex techniques, thereby increasing their risks of infection with HIV and other sexually transmitted diseases.[28]

Elder's Drinking Habits

Studies suggest that Americans ≥65 drink less heavily than their juniors. Explanations for this finding include:

1. By the time they reach 65, many adults have resolved their addiction problems.
2. Many alcohol-dependent persons die before reaching age 65.
3. Physiologic factors change. (*See Blood Alcohol Concentration, Chapter 4.*)
4. Elders may have poorer recall, or experience difficulty answering computational questions included in routine alcohol screening.
5. Physiologic effects of alcohol may be mistakenly attributed to the aging process, chronic disease, or side effects of prescription medications.
6. Household surveys may not include nursing-home residents with alcohol disorders.[2,27]

Race/Ethnicity Factors

Table 4 data show that, during 1995, an estimated 34.0% of American White males used alcohol for ≥51 days, compared with 26.9% of African American males and 26.6% of Hispanic males. Much greater differences are seen among female racial/ethnic groups: an estimated 16.9% of White females used alcohol for ≥51 days, compared with 10.7% of African American females and only 5.4% of Hispanic females.[22]

> All racial and ethnic groups comprise subgroups with different backgrounds and cultural drinking practices.

For all racial and ethnic groups, data on alcohol consumption are complex and often conflicting, because each group comprises subgroups with different backgrounds and cultural drinking practices; e.g., drinking practices vary greatly among Native American tribal groups. Caetano[29] found that a higher percentage of Mexican Americans report alcohol problems than the percentage of other Hispanic groups in the United States; Mexican Americans also have more liberal attitudes towards drinking.

Suddendorf[30] reports that Asian Americans may limit their drinking because, upon ingestion of alcohol, some subgroups experience a highly visible facial flush, accompanied by other symptoms of discomfort. (*See Metabolism, Chapter 4.*) However, Chi et al.[31] report that certain Asian American subgroups have consumption rates approaching that of the U.S. population as a whole.[27]

Emergencies and Deaths

Alcohol use often results in injuries, accidental or intentional. In a study of 16,251 patients admitted to the RAC Shock Trauma Center in Baltimore, Maryland, from July 1987—June 1993, Champion et al.[32] found that 36% of the men and 20% of the women had positive BACs. Forty percent of these drinkers were 21 to 35 years of age, 42% were motorcycle drivers or passengers, 41% were injured pedestrians, and 40% were victims of intentional violence (assault, gunshot, or knife wounds). Champion et al. report similar findings at many other U.S. trauma centers.[33]

> Drinkers often abuse other drugs, particularly heroin/morphine and cocaine.

Drinkers often abuse other drugs. Of the estimated 531,800 emergency-room drug abuse episodes reported to the Drug Abuse Warning Network (DAWN) during 1995, 32% involved persons who had used alcohol in combination with another drug.[34] Of the 8,541 drug abuse deaths reported to DAWN during 1993 by medical examiners, approximately 40.3% were caused by concurrent use of alcohol and another drug; the second drug in about 52% of the cases was heroin/morphine, and, in about 46% of the cases, cocaine.[35] (*See also Alcohol and Illegal Drugs, Chapter 11.*)

As discussed in Chapter 1, a significant number of traffic fatalities, drownings, and homicides are associated with alcohol use. Physiologic disorders, particularly liver cirrhosis, account for other alcohol-related deaths. (*See Chapter 10.*) Approximately 5% of all deaths in the United States involve alcohol.[2]

Quick Facts Epidemiologic Data

NIAAA manages the Quick Facts electronic bulletin board, which enables anyone with a computer and modem to access statistics on alcohol abuse and dependence. Quick Facts uses a bulletin board system (BBS) software package and does not require an on-line fee, although out-of-area users must pay long-distance telephone charges. Quick Facts may be accessed using the following specifications: BBS number: 202-289-4112 (in the United States).

On the World Wide Web, Quick Facts is available at *telnet.fedworld.gov* and *www.fedworld.gov*:

1. *telnet.fedworld.gov*—select 1 FEDWORLD, enter your first and last name, select D for Health Safety and Nutrition Mall, select 1 for Health Gateway Systems, then press Q and select #118 for Quick Facts

2. *www.fedworld.gov*—select FEDWORLD TELNET SITE from information listing, enter your first and last name, and proceed as directed above.

Chapter Summary

1. Researchers obtain epidemiological data on alcohol use and misuse, and their consequences, via surveillance and survey research.

2. After repeal of Prohibition in 1933, per capita alcohol consumption increased, fluctuating periodically, until peaking in 1981 at just below 2.8 gallons of pure alcohol per year.

3. Studies of alcohol use have consistently found that men drink more than women and experience more adverse consequences.

4. Increases in heavy drinking by females have been found within certain subgroups, e.g., college students and women working in nontraditional, male-dominated occupations.

5. Binge drinking, having ≥5 drinks at one sitting, is widespread on many American college campuses.

6. Because all racial and ethnic groups comprise subgroups with different backgrounds and cultural drinking practices, data on alcohol consumption are complex and often conflicting.

7. Trauma center data show that alcohol use immediately prior to injury is common among persons 21 to 35 years of age, motorcycle drivers or passengers, injured pedestrians, and victims of intentional violence.

8. During 1993, approximately 40.3% of drug abuse deaths reported to DAWN involved concurrent use of alcohol and another drug; most of the decedents had combined alcohol with either heroin/morphine or cocaine.

Progress Test A (Chapters 1 & 2)

1. Fermentation, which produces alcohol, occurs naturally when airborne _____ act on substances containing sugar.

2. The _____ amendment to the Constitution, passed in 1919, established national Prohibition.

3. Prohibition failed because many Americans considered it an intolerable infringement of _____ _____.

4. In 1988, Congress passed Public Law 100-960, which requires that alcoholic beverage containers carry a _____ label.

5. U.S. alcohol-related _____ _____ _____ cost an estimated $46 billion annually.

6. Men drink _____ than women and experience _____ adverse consequences.

7. College students who binge drink may experience _____ _____, act aggressively, and drive after drinking.

8. Physiologic effects of alcohol, in older patients, may be mistakenly attributed to the aging process, chronic disease, or _____ _____ of prescription medications.

9. Of the estimated 531,800 emergency-room drug abuse episodes reported to DAWN during 1995, 32% involved persons who had used alcohol ____ _____ with another drug.

Chapter 3   Theories on Alcohol Misuse

Although researchers have long tried to determine why people misuse alcohol, scientists are still only beginning to understand the problem. Most studies have focused on the drinking habits of men, but recent studies have included both sexes.

> People may drink as a result of one influence or overlapping combinations of influences.

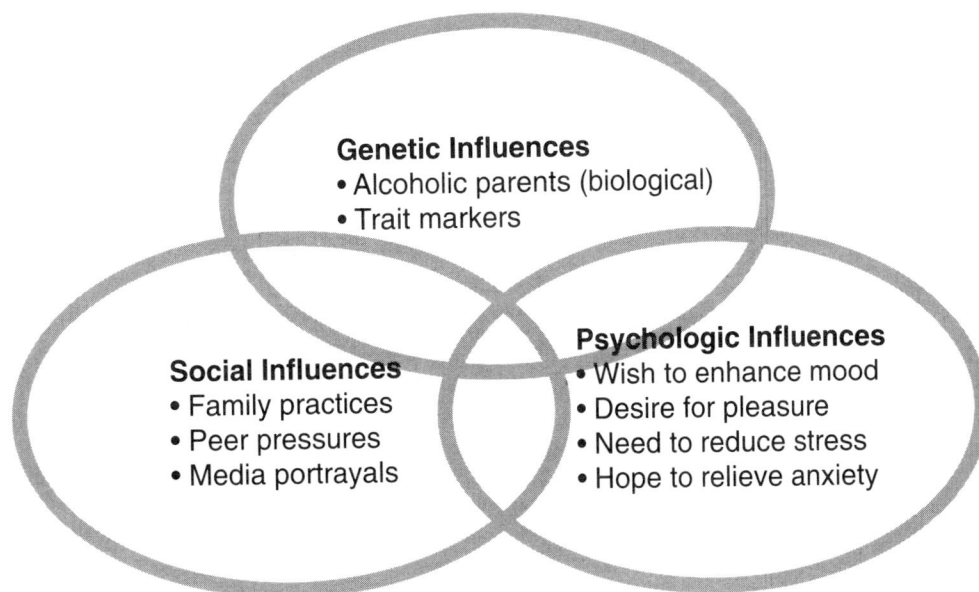

This chapter explains current theories by reviewing genetic, psychologic, and social influences associated with alcohol misuse. As Fig. 3 shows, people may drink as a result of one influence or overlapping combinations of influences.

Genetic Influences
- Alcoholic parents (biological)
- Trait markers

Social Influences
- Family practices
- Peer pressures
- Media portrayals

Psychologic Influences
- Wish to enhance mood
- Desire for pleasure
- Need to reduce stress
- Hope to relieve anxiety

Fig. 3. Influences Associated With Alcohol Misuse

Genetic Influences

Whether alcohol abuse and dependence can be inherited has been the subject of many studies.

Adoption Studies

Several studies indicate that children born to alcoholic parents, but adopted away soon after birth by nonrelatives, had a greater risk for alcohol dependence than adopted-away children born to nonalcoholic parents. A review of adoption study data by Merikangas[36] suggests that, in general, persons with an alcoholic biological parent have about a 2.5-fold increased general risk for alcohol dependence, regardless of their home environment.[2]

Based on a study of a large group of Swedish adoptees, Cloninger[37] proposed dividing "alcoholism" (alcohol dependence) into the two types described in Table 6.[38] Researchers have found that age of onset is an important distinguishing factor: the earlier onset Type II alcohol dependence is associated not only with greater genetic risk, but with more severe alcohol-related social problems (e.g., criminality and other antisocial behaviors).[39]

Table 6. Cloninger's Types of Alcohol Dependence	
Types	**Patients' Characteristics/Circumstances**

Type I	These alcohol-dependent persons:
	• Lose control of their drinking after age 25 (late onset alcohol dependence)
	• Are influenced more by environmental drinking stimuli than by heredity
	• Possess passive-dependent personality traits, including:
	  • Low levels of novelty seeking (inflexibility; contemplative behavior)
	  • High levels of reward dependence (inhibited behavior)
	  • High levels of harm avoidance (concern about reactions of others)

Type II	These alcohol-dependent persons:
	• Lose control of their drinking before age 25 (early onset alcohol dependence)
	• Are influenced more by heredity than by environmental factors
	• Behave in a manner consistent with an antisocial personality, which includes:
	  • High levels of novelty seeking (impulsivity and excitability)
	  • Low levels of reward dependence (distant social relations)
	  • Low levels of harm avoidance (uninhibited and brash behavior)

Twin Studies

Several researchers have compared the existence of alcohol dependence in pairs of identical twins (identical genetically), and pairs of fraternal twins (no more genetically alike than non-twin siblings).

Cadoret's review[40] of 13 studies showed a greater concordance for drinking behavior and alcohol dependence among identical twins, even when they lived apart, than among fraternal twins. McGue et al.,[41] in a more recent twin study, suggest that genetic influences contribute significantly to early onset alcohol dependence in males, but only moderately to late onset alcohol dependence in males and alcohol-related disorders in females.[2]

Trait Markers

Table 7 shows selected genetic trait markers which have been evaluated in preliminary studies and which may be associated with susceptibility to alcohol dependence.[2] (*See also Biological State Markers, Table 15, Chapter 6.*)

Table 7. Trait Markers of Vulnerability to Alcohol Misuse	
Potential Markers	**Selected Study Results**
Beta activity	• Davis et al.[42] found that resting-state EEGs in sober, awake alcoholics contained excess beta activity • Ehlers and Schuckit[43] showed that men aged 18 to 25 years with alcohol-dependent fathers displayed significantly more beta activity after consuming alcohol than did control subjects with nonalcoholic fathers.
Platelet uptake of serotonin	Rausch et al.[44] showed a higher rate of platelet serotonin uptake in men with alcohol-dependent fathers, compared with control subjects.
Prolactin and cortisol in blood	Schuckit et al.[45,46] showed that, after moderate alcohol consumption, males with alcohol-dependent fathers have decreased blood levels of the hormones prolactin and cortisol; these drinkers report less severe alcohol effects, compared with control subjects.
Baseline heart rate	Finn and Pihl[47] found that the baseline heart rate of males with multigenerational family histories of male alcohol dependence increased significantly within 20 minutes of ingestion of a relatively large amount of alcohol.

Researchers are trying to identify the specific genes which carry susceptibility to alcohol dependence. In 1990, Blum et al.[48] reported higher-than-normal prevalence of the A1 allele in brain tissue taken from 35 deceased advanced alcoholics; the A1 allele belongs to the dopamine D2 receptor gene located on chromosome 11. However, subsequent work by several other researchers did not link this gene with alcohol dependence, but suggested that the A1 allele might interact with or modify the effect of other genes, thereby leading to the disorder.[2]

Psychologic Influences

Psychologic influences related to alcohol misuse include cognitive processes (e.g., thinking, attention, and memory) and affective aspects (e.g., feelings and attitudes).[2] Marlatt[49] summed it up when he suggested that alcohol is often perceived as a "magic elixir," capable of promoting social skills, sexual pleasure, confidence, power, and aggression. The following section gives results of some research on psychologic influences.

Enhancing Mood

Alcohol is a disinhibitor at every level of brain functioning, affecting behavior and conscience. Alcohol narrows one's focus of attention, thereby decreasing internal conflict. It blocks inhibitions, making social behaviors more spontaneous and extreme when stimuli are compelling. Steele and Josephs[50] hypothesize that, when inhibitions are blocked and internal conflict is reduced, self-images may inflate, leading to feelings of power and control—which some persons seek to achieve through drinking.[2]

Roy stares into a juror's eyes and says: "This man is innocent; that can be your only verdict!" Defense attorney Roy glows in this moment of power; the prosecution failed to present enough evidence against his client. Roy himself isn't convinced his client is innocent, but such doubts don't bother him now; his usual three swigs of bourbon before he entered the courtroom have dispelled them, allowing him to present a dynamic summation.

Obtaining Pleasure

Many people drink because, as their BAC increases and they become intoxicated, they feel happier. However, as their bodies metabolize the alcohol, decreasing their BAC, their feelings of pleasure often change to extreme sadness.

Another Saturday night and, as usual, 58-year-old Vera sits alone, watching TV and sipping sherry. The first couple of glasses give her feelings of warmth and pleasure, and she forgets her loneliness. Two hours—and three fourths of a bottle—later, Vera wipes the tears from her eyes and staggers to bed, praying she will sleep the whole night. As a rule, she awakens after a few hours to toss and turn fitfully, plagued by unhappy memories.

Research indicates that people differ in the degree of pleasure they derive from drinking. Newlin and Thomson[51] report that males with alcohol-dependent parents may experience enhanced pleasure as their BAC increases, and diminished anxiety and depression as their BAC decreases. Some researchers believe such responses to alcohol may characterize <u>any</u> persons at high risk for alcohol dependence.[2]

Managing Stress

Many drinkers have learned that alcohol consumption reduces anxiety, at least temporarily. Sher[52] reports that alcohol does this by dampening patients' stress response. Therefore, if alcohol is especially helpful in times of stress, a person might continue to use it to manage a particular stressor.[2]

> *Robert gulps down another shot of whiskey, while his wife, at the front door, calls for him to hurry, so they won't be late for dinner at her mother's house. Each Sunday, he humors his wife by going there, but he hates it. The old bitch does nothing but criticize him from the time he arrives until he leaves; even worse, she doesn't allow liquor in the house—so, each week, he tanks up, on an empty stomach, before leaving home.*

Fulfilling Expectations

Expectations, like other beliefs, represent stored memories of experiences and observations; e.g., sexual activities are a common focus of people's expectations. Leigh's[53] studies showed that, compared with persons who drank moderately, both males and females who drank heavily had stronger expectations concerning three of alcohol's effects: increased sexual desire, decreased nervousness, and increased risk taking. The highest level of drinking occurred among women who had strong expectations about alcohol's effects and negative attitudes toward sex—who felt nervous or guilty. That these women may use alcohol to reduce their sexual inhibitions is supported by findings that many people use alcohol before having sex for the first time or the first time with a new partner.[54]

> *When her dinner partner touches her hand and suggests they go to her apartment to make love, Ruby quickly takes another sip of Chablis. She is sorry she agreed to this first date with him, for the expensive restaurant's sumptuous food and romantic music are creating no sexual chemistry for her. As the evening wears on, and the waiter refills her glass for the fourth time, Ruby begins to feel mellow. She gently squeezes her partner's hand; understanding the signal, he says, "Let's go, now." As they leave the restaurant, Ruby realizes that her nervousness and guilty feelings about having sex with him have disappeared.*

Social Influences

The most important social influences related to alcohol consumption are direct interactions with others, particularly family members and peers.

Family Practices

Studies indicate that offspring alcohol use does not always correspond with parental use (e.g., Harburg et al.[55] found that adolescents were less likely to imitate their parents' drinking when it became extreme; Barnes et al.[56] found that adolescents drank heavily even though they had abstaining mothers). Kandel and Andrews[57] found, however, that, in initial use of alcohol by adolescents, parents played a significant role, both through their own alcohol use and through their attitudes toward its harmful effects. Ringwalt and Palmer[58] found that African American adolescents were significantly more apt than White adolescents to understand the adverse health consequences of drinking alcohol and to be concerned about parental disapproval (the Whites were more concerned about peer disapproval).[2]

> Offspring alcohol use does not always correspond with parental use.

Kandel and Andrews[57] found that teenagers' perceived closeness to parents discouraged teenagers' drinking, and Barnes et al.[56] found that adolescents whose parents provided high levels of nurturing and support reported fewer alcohol-related problem behaviors than did youths who received low levels of these parenting practices. Holmes and Robins[59] found that parental discipline described as unfair, harsh, and inconsistent was predictive of alcohol and depressive disorders in their children during adulthood. Thus, parenting practices may play a role in alcohol misuse throughout life.[2]

> *Fourteen-year-old Jeremiah sits on the couch, drinking beer out of a large mug, in the apartment of some new friends. He feels safe here, and, even though he doesn't really like the taste of beer, it helps him forget his father, who gets violently drunk every night. His father doesn't care about him; all he does is beat up on him. His new friends care about him, though. They buy his beer for him, since he doesn't have an ID to prove he's 21. They tell him he should quit school, get a job, and move in with them. That sure would teach his father a lesson!*

Peer Pressures

The most powerful predictor of alcohol use among young people is peer pressure (e.g., friends using alcohol and other drugs, and friends preventing a youth from using them). The closeness of the peer relationship also affects drinking behavior: Morgan and Grube[60] found that adolescents are more likely to continue their alcohol use if a best friend drinks.[2] Several studies indicate that college students generally overestimate the amount of alcohol their peers drink; these inaccurate perceptions can increase their own consumption.[28]

Peer pressure is not limited to young people. Alexander and Duff[61] found that, in some retirement communities, peer pressure to increase alcohol intake may contribute to late onset alcohol dependence in older people, which is rarely associated with a family history of alcohol dependence or psychologic disorders.[2]

> *Norman and Milly love their new apartment in a Florida retirement community. He is making friends and playing golf three times a week; she is enjoying her afternoon bridge games. The fun really begins at the cocktail hour by the pool each day; here, as Norman and Milly have discovered, they feel happy, and, after two or three martinis, more like eating dinner. Drinking has never been a part of their lifestyle during 40 years of marriage; if they don't drink now, however, their new friends tease them, calling them prudes. So they figure, "Why not join the crowd and live a little?"*

Media Portrayals

Limited information is available about how, or if, media presentations motivate drinking. In an analysis of the portrayals of alcohol drinking in U.S. prime-time fictional TV broadcasts, Wallach et al.[62] found, in half of the episodes, an average of eight drinking acts per hour, by characters generally depicted as of high social status. In only 10% of the episodes were alcohol problems clearly presented.[2]

Chapter Summary

1. A patient's alcohol misuse may be influenced by genetic, social, and/or psychologic influences.

2. Adoption studies indicate that children born to alcoholic parents, but adopted away soon after birth by nonrelatives, had a greater risk for alcohol dependence than adopted-away children born to nonalcoholic parents.

3. Cloninger divides alcohol dependence into two types; of these, Type II alcohol dependence is associated with greater genetic risk and more severe alcohol-related social problems.

4. Twin studies showed a greater concordance for drinking behavior and alcohol dependence among identical twins, even when they lived apart, than among fraternal twins.

5. Genetic trait markers which may be associated with susceptibility to alcohol dependence include beta activity, platelet uptake of serotonin, prolactin and cortisol in blood, and baseline heart rate.

6. Marlatt suggested that alcohol is commonly perceived as a "magic elixir."

7. Because alcohol blocks inhibitions, it makes social behavior more spontaneous and extreme when stimuli are compelling.

8. Any persons at high risk for alcohol dependence may experience greater pleasure during periods of increasing BAC and fewer unpleasant effects during decreasing BAC.

9. If people find drinking especially helpful in times of stress, they might continue to use it to manage a particular stressor.

10. African American adolescents are significantly more apt than Whites to appreciate the adverse health consequences of drinking alcohol and to be concerned about parental disapproval.

11. The most powerful predictor of alcohol use among young people is peer pressure.

Chapter 4   Physiologic Aspects of Alcohol Consumption

The only beverage alcohol is ethanol, or ethyl alcohol, which, in this course, is referred to as alcohol.

As a first step in evaluating whether patients are misusing alcohol, health care workers need an understanding of how it affects patients. Alcohols, which abound in nature, include cholesterol, menthol, isopropyl alcohol, ethylene glycol, and methanol. However, the only beverage alcohol is ethanol, or ethyl alcohol, which, in this course, is referred to as alcohol.

Alcoholic Beverages

Beverage alcohol is produced by fermentation, when yeasts of the genus *Saccharomyces* break down sugar molecules. Yeast on the skins of crushed grapes breaks down the sugars to produce the alcohol of table wines (e.g., Chablis, rosé, Chianti); when yeast is added to wort (water and crushed grains whose starch has been enzymatically transformed into sugar), the end product is ale or beer. Alcohol production ceases when the yeasts die: some species succumb to an alcohol level of 5%; other yeasts can tolerate levels as high as 15% or 16%.[63,64,65] To produce fortified wines (e.g., port and sherry), wine makers add alcohol during or after fermentation; to produce higher-alcohol-content beers (ice-brewed), brewers lower the water temperature to below freezing, which allows slightly longer yeast survival and fermentation.

A bottle of whiskey containing about 60% water and 40% alcohol is labeled 80 proof, which represents twice the alcohol concentration by volume.

The making of spirits, or "hard" liquor (e.g., whiskey and vodka), requires enzymatic conversion of grain or potato starch to sugar, addition of yeast for fermentation, and distillation of the resulting alcohol. This process produces pure alcohol, which is then blended with water, bottled, and sold as liquors with specific proofs; e.g., a bottle of whiskey containing about 60% water and 40% alcohol is labeled 80 proof, which represents twice the alcohol concentration by volume.[64,65,66] The term proof evolved from a 17th century English custom of proving at least a 57% alcohol content (114 proof). The procedure involved moistening gunpowder with a beverage, then applying a flame; a beverage containing at least 57% alcohol would ignite and be called "proof spirits."[63]

Alcoholic beverages also contain congeners, secondary products of fermentation, which provide taste, smell, and color. Congeners, such as tannic acid and furfural, are released by the wooden barrels in which alcoholic beverages are aged.[65] Goodwin[63] says that Russian vodka sometimes contains considerable amounts of wood alcohol (methanol). The amount of methanol in one serving of vodka is small, but, with several drinks, the amount multiplies; consuming 1 ounce of methanol has been fatal. This poisonous substance can also cause blindness; Goodwin recommends that manufacturers list the congener content on containers, just as ingredients are listed on food packages.

Calculating Alcohol Intake

> Drinkers often fool themselves when they say: "It's only a beer, not a real drink."

Table 8 compares the amount of pure (or absolute) alcohol ingested per serving of various alcoholic beverages. Drinkers often fool themselves when they say: "It's only a beer, not a real drink." As Table 8 shows, drinking one 12-ounce can of most beers represents the <u>same</u>—or a <u>greater</u>—intake of pure alcohol as drinking 1.5 ounces of bourbon or gin.

U.S. beverage preferences are changing, as shown in Fig. 4 (these data were calculated using the same methods and beverage sales statistics as Fig. 2 data). Consumption of beer and wine remained fairly level during the 22-year period, but hard liquor use decreased considerably.[2,20,21]

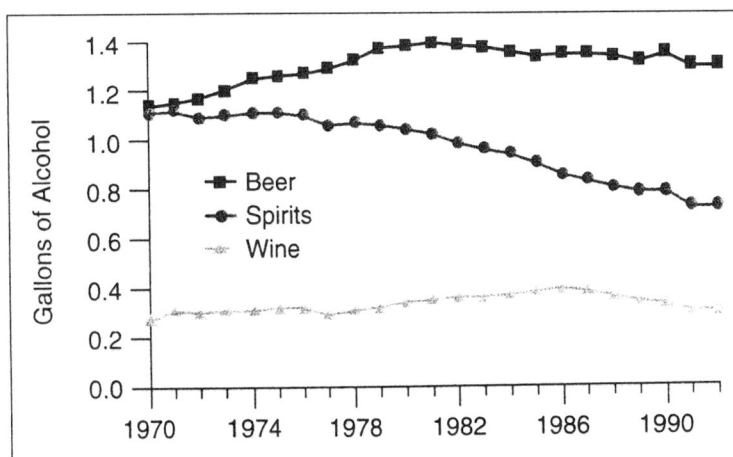

Fig. 4. Beverage Preferences, U.S., 1970-1992: average per capita consumption of pure alcohol by beverage type

Table 8. Calculation of Pure Alcohol Intake

Alcoholic Beverages	Percent Alcohol	Usual Serving	Ergo: Pure Alcohol Intake is:*
Beers:			
• Budweiser Light®	4.2	12 oz	0.50 oz
• Miller Lite®	4.5	12 oz	0.54 oz
• Bud Dry®, Busch®	4.9	12 oz	0.59 oz
• Budweiser®, Michelob®, Miller Beer®, Miller Draft®	5.0	12 oz	0.60 oz
• Bud Ice®, Red Wolf®	5.5	12 oz	0.66 oz
• Michelob Malt®	5.8	12 oz	0.70 oz
• Miller Life Ice®	5.9	12 oz	0.71 oz
• Magnum®	5.9	12 oz	0.71 oz
• Samuel Adams Triple Bock®	17.0	8 oz	1.36 oz
Table Wines (unfortified):			
• Boone's Sangria®	7.5	4 oz	0.30 oz
• Riunite Lambrusco®	8.0	4 oz	0.32 oz
• Sutter Home White Zinfandel®	9.0	4 oz	0.36 oz
• Blue Nun 1995 Liebfraumilch Rheinhessen®	9.5	4 oz	0.38 oz
• Carlo Rossi Blush®	9.5	4 oz	0.38 oz
• Almaden Blush Chablis®	11.0	4 oz	0.44 oz
• Taylor Lake Country White®	11.0	4 oz	0.44 oz
• Chateau Morrisette Virginia White Reisling®	12.0	4 oz	0.48 oz
• Chianti Ruffino 1994®	12.0	4 oz	0.48 oz
• Glenn Allen Merlot 1994®	12.5	4 oz	0.50 oz
• Louis Jardot 1995 Beaujolais-Villages Jardot®	12.5	4 oz	0.50 oz
• Sutter Home California Sauvignon Blanc®	13.0	4 oz	0.52 oz
• Ernest & Julio Gallo Cabernet Sauvignon®	13.0	4 oz	0.52 oz
• Beringer Chardonnay®	13.4	4 oz	0.54 oz
Wines (fortified):			
• Harveys Bristol Dry Sherry®	17.5	3 oz	0.53 oz
• Martini & Rossi Extra Dry Vermouth®	18.0	3 oz	0.54 oz
• Sandeman Port®	19.0	3 oz	0.57 oz
Liqueurs (distilled):			
• Baileys Irish Creme®	17.0	1.5 oz	0.26 oz
• Kahlúa®	26.5	1.5 oz	0.40 oz
• Grand Marnier®	40.0	1.5 oz	0.60 oz
Spirits or Hard Liquors (distilled):			
• Beefeater London Distilled Dry Gin®	40.0	1.5 oz	0.60 oz
• Jim Beam Bourbon®	40.0	1.5 oz	0.60 oz
• Johnnie Walker Black Label Scotch Whiskey®	40.0	1.5 oz	0.60 oz
• Montezuma Aztec Gold Tequila®	40.0	1.5 oz	0.60 oz
• Myers's Original Dark Jamaican Rum®	40.0	1.5 oz	0.60 oz
• Pierre Smirnoff Vodka®	40.0	1.5 oz	0.60 oz
• Bacardi Superior Light-Dry Puerto Rican Rum®	40.0	1.5 oz	0.60 oz
• White Label Dewar's Scotch Whiskey®	40.0	1.5 oz	0.60 oz
• Smirnoff #57 Vodka®	50.0	1.5 oz	0.75 oz
• Bacardi Superior Rum®	75.5	1.5 oz	1.13 oz

* Pure alcohol intake is calculated by multiplying the % alcohol by the usual serving.

Note: Some sources use 5 oz., instead of 4 oz., as the usual serving of wine, thereby increasing alcohol intake.

Alcohol Absorption and Metabolism

The body metabolizes most ingested alcohol. Only 2% to 10% is exhaled via the respiratory system or excreted in urine or sweat.[67]

Absorption

Although most alcohol is absorbed through the small intestine and metabolized by the liver, other organs do play a role. The oral and esophageal mucosa absorb a small amount, diffusing it into the bloodstream. Then, in the stomach, a small amount of the alcohol is absorbed, and at least two gastric alcohol dehydrogenase (ADH) enzymes metabolize a limited amount. When drinkers take aspirin, cimetidine (Tagamet®), or ranitidine (Zantac®), these medications reduce gastric ADH, resulting in higher BACs.[68]

Alcohol not metabolized or absorbed in the stomach moves into the small intestine, where most absorption and diffusion occur. The rate of this absorption determines BAC. Table 9 shows some factors affecting this rate.[63,67]

Table 9. Factors Affecting Alcohol Absorption	
Quicker absorption when:	• The stomach is empty, and alcohol does not have to compete with larger food molecules to cross gastric mucosa. • The small intestine is empty, and the stomach can empty rapidly. • Stomach contents are carbonated (e.g., champagne, sparkling wines, drinks mixed with carbonated soda).
Slower absorption when:	• There are proteins, fats, and carbohydrates in the stomach, which compete with alcohol to cross mucosa. • There are proteins and fats in the stomach, which delay stomach emptying time. • Gastric emptying is delayed due to the presence of food in the small intestine.

When the concentration of alcohol in the blood reaches that in the stomach or small intestine, absorption stops. Any remaining alcohol or additional intake stays in these organs until BAC decreases enough for absorption to resume.[68] BAC decrease depends, primarily, on hepatic metabolism.

Metabolism

The bloodstream transports most ingested alcohol to the liver, where it is ultimately converted to acetic acid (the acid of vinegar). Alcohol metabolism occurs at a relatively constant rate, averaging about 1 ounce of pure alcohol per 3 hours, for adults.[69]

Figs. 5 and 6 illustrate the <u>primary</u> pathway of alcohol metabolism. In a liver cell, alcohol is converted to toxic acetaldehyde by hepatic ADH enzymes, of which there are several kinds. Acetaldehyde, in turn, is metabolized by another enzyme, aldehyde dehydrogenase (ALDH), to acetic acid.[2] At each of these steps, the oxidized form of nicotinamide adenine dinucleotide (NAD^+) is converted to a reduced form (NADH), which, in excess, causes a number of metabolic derangements, including inhibition of fatty-acid oxidation.[70]

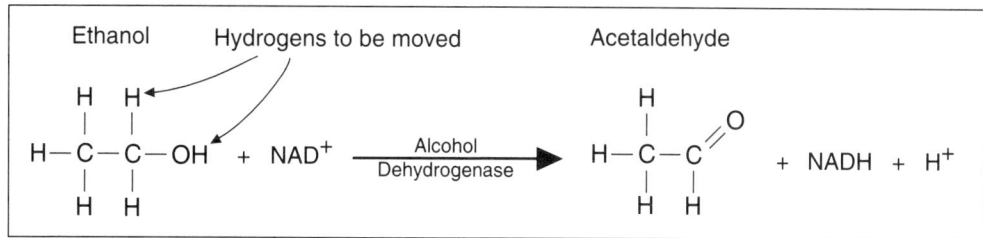

Fig. 5. Molecular View of the First Step in Alcohol Metabolism: Ethanol, converted to acetaldehyde in the presence of alcohol dehydrogenase (ADH), loses two of its hydrogen atoms, one of them to NAD^+.

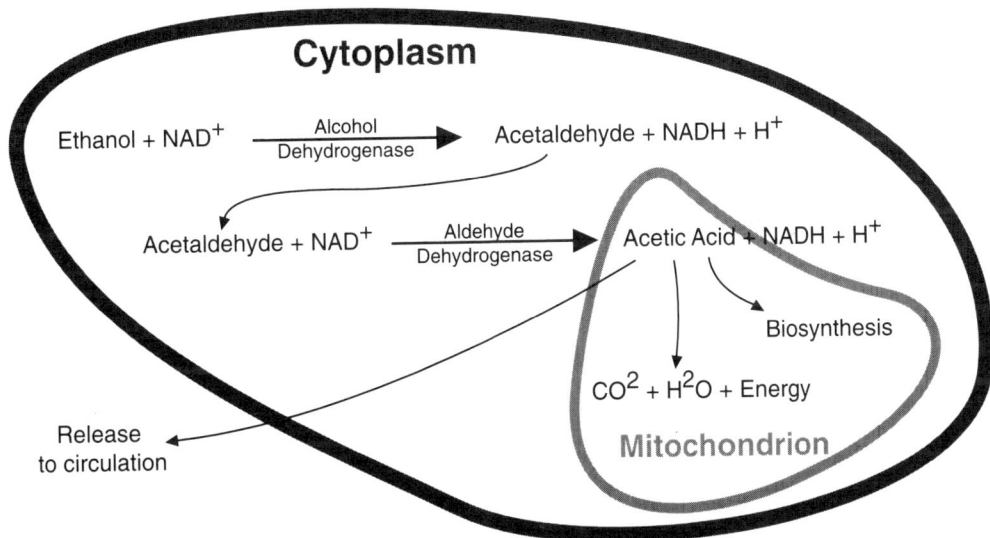

Fig. 6. Metabolism in the Liver Cell of a Nonalcoholic: First, the alcohol-to-acetaldehyde conversion occurs in the cytoplasm (see also molecular view, Fig. 5). Then, another enzyme, aldehyde dehydrogenase, converts acetaldehyde to acetic acid. Each of these steps produces a molecule of NADH. Within the cell's mitochondria (one shown above), acetic acid is directed toward different pathways, depending on the energy needs of the liver cell.

The relative concentrations of NAD$^+$ and NADH determine the fate of the acetic acid; it may be:

1. Metabolized further to yield energy, carbon dioxide (CO_2) and water (H_2O), if the NAD$^+$/NADH ratio is low
2. Used for the synthesis of other molecules, if the NAD$^+$/NADH ratio is high
3. Released into the circulation for use by other tissues.[2]

Secondary pathways of alcohol metabolism in a liver cell are (1) the microsomal ethanol-oxidizing system (MEOS), and (2) the catalase system. Both pathways yield acetaldehyde, which is then converted to acetic acid, but they appear to function only when concentrations of alcohol are high. MEOS contains the enzyme cytochrome P-4502E1, which has an extraordinary capacity to convert certain anesthetic agents (e.g., enflurane), medications (e.g., isoniazid), and analgesic agents (e.g., acetaminophen) into toxic metabolites.[2,70]

> One genetic variant of mitochondrial ALDH appears in some American Asian subgroups.

The liver contains four distinct ALDH enzymes. One genetic variant of mitochondrial ALDH, arising from a single amino acid substitution, appears in some American Asian subgroups. Enzyme activity is drastically reduced, which can result in circulating acetaldehyde levels 10 to 20 times higher than those in persons who produce active ALDH. The effects of high acetaldehyde levels include facial flush, palpitations, dizziness, and nausea.[2]

Blood Alcohol Concentration

BAC is the weight of alcohol in a specific volume of blood, expressed in g/dL. (*See Table 3, Chapter 1, for equivalencies.*) Although BAC fluctuates with the alcohol absorption and metabolism rates, as previously discussed, it is also related to gender, weight, and lean body mass.

Alcohol, which is distributed throughout total body water (about 42 liters for a 70-kg person), is more soluble in water than in fat. Therefore, BAC produced by a given volume of alcohol is higher in women than in men because:

1. Women normally have smaller bodies through which to distribute the alcohol.

2. Compared with men, women tend to have proportionately more fatty tissue (which requires a minimal blood supply), less muscle tissue (which requires a hefty blood supply), and, therefore, a diminished need for body water and blood supply, which would dilute the alcohol.[6,24,71]

In both genders, age-related increases in the ratio of body fat to lean muscle mass result in higher BACs for elders consuming the same amount of alcohol as they did when they were younger.[2]

Fig. 7 compares the BACs for a 140-lb. male and a 120-lb. female ingesting the same amounts of pure alcohol over a 1-hour period.[2] As shown, a female consuming three drinks in 1 hour has a BAC of 0.11 g/dL, which is just over the legal limit (0.10 g/dL) defining intoxication in most states, and is far above the 0.08 g/dL limit in about a dozen states. (*See Motor Vehicle Crashes, Chapter 1.*)

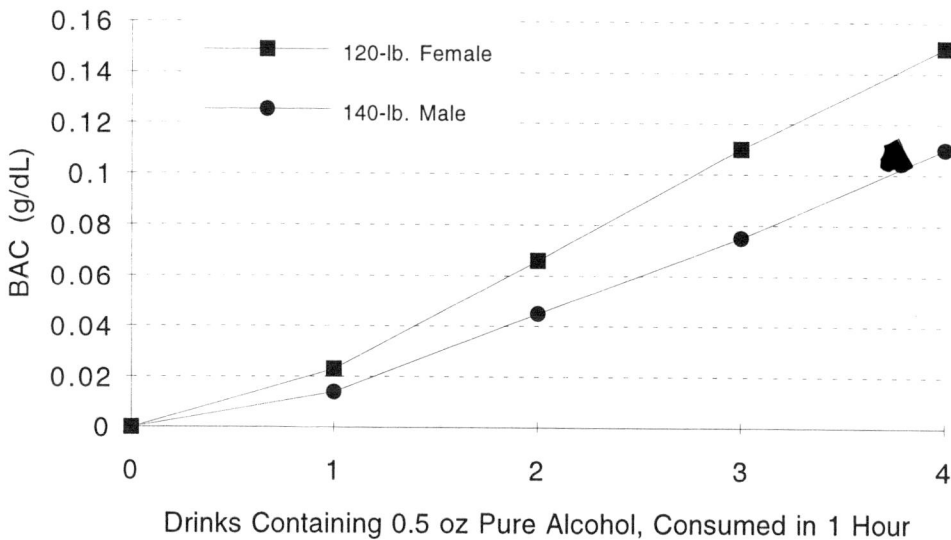

Fig. 7. BAC Comparison—120-lb. Female and 140-lb. Male: BAC increases faster in women than in men because of gender differences in body fat, water, and size.

Drinks Containing 0.5 oz Pure Alcohol, Consumed in 1 Hour

Effects of Alcohol

Effects of alcohol on the central nervous system (CNS) and body support systems vary according to BAC. Table 10 shows typical psychologic and physiologic effects of alcohol consumption, as BAC increases.[2,72] Many chronic drinkers with tolerance to alcohol (*see Chapter 5*) may not exhibit some of the effects, even at BACs which would prove lethal for drinkers who have not developed tolerance.[73] However, clinicians evaluating patients experiencing the effects listed in Table 10 must determine their true causes, because some can result from serious medical disorders, e.g.:

1. Incoordination and impaired judgment associated with alcohol intoxication can resemble signs and symptoms of certain general illnesses, such as multiple sclerosis and diabetic acidosis.[74]
2. Profound coma in the presence of relatively low BACs might be caused by a complicating illness, such as meningitis, pneumonia, head injury, or portal-systemic encephalopathy.[75]

Table 10. Typical Effects of Alcohol Consumption		
Intoxication Level	BAC (g/dL)	Findings: Psychologic/Physiologic
Mild	0.030 to 0.049	More talkative than usual; euphoria in drinkers who have not developed tolerance to alcohol
	0.050 to 0.059	Impaired attention and vigilance; relaxation; tranquillity; sedation; lowered inhibitions in drinkers without tolerance to alcohol
	0.060 to 0.099	Unsteadiness when standing; lack of coordination; dizziness; impaired sense of smell and taste; elevated pain threshold; mild euphoria; loud, profuse talking; self-satisfaction; impaired judgment
Moderate	0.100 to 0.149	Staggering when blindfolded; impaired short-term memory ("blackout"); inability to do math calculations; poorer performance in sensory and motor activities; mood swings, shifting from laughter to tears and rage
	0.150 to 0.199	Staggering even without being blindfolded; slurred speech; slow reaction time; increased impairment of mental and motor activities; erratic emotions
	0.200 to 0.249	Marked clumsiness; pylorospasm; nausea and vomiting
Severe	0.250 to 0.299	Some loss of consciousness; nystagmus
	0.300 to 0.399	Labored breathing; subject to hypothermia and amnesia
	0.400 to 0.459	Alcoholic coma: low body temperature, depressed respiration, almost imperceptible pulse, markedly decreased or absent reflexes
	≥0.460[81]	Death (in 50% of patients, BACs of 0.50 g/dL are lethal)[83]

People with mild to moderate intoxication need no immediate care. (*See Chapter 10 for treatment of severe intoxication.*) A patient with a BAC of 0.15 g/dL, who stops drinking, will reach 0 BAC in about 10 hours (on average, BAC falls by 0.015 g/dL per hour). As the patient's BAC starts to decrease, signs and symptoms of withdrawal may appear. Many drinkers withdraw from alcohol on their own; however, serious withdrawal signs and symptoms justify hospitalization. (*See Withdrawal and Medical Detoxification, Chapter 12.*)

On average, BAC falls by 0.015 g/dL per hour.

Chapter Summary

1. The only beverage alcohol is ethanol, or ethyl alcohol, which, in this course, is referred to as alcohol.

2. Beverage alcohol is produced by fermentation, when yeasts of the genus *Saccharomyces* break down sugar molecules.

3. Drinking one 12-ounce can of most beers represents the same—or a greater—intake of pure alcohol as drinking 1.5 ounces of bourbon or gin.

4. Alcohol not metabolized or absorbed in the stomach moves into the small intestine, where most absorption and diffusion occur.

5. The bloodstream transports most ingested alcohol to the liver, where it is ultimately converted to acetic acid.

6. Alcohol metabolism occurs at a relatively constant rate, averaging about 1 ounce of pure alcohol per 3 hours, for adults.

7. BAC produced by a given volume of alcohol is higher in women than in men because:

    a. Women normally have smaller bodies through which to distribute the alcohol, and
    b. Women tend to have proportionately more fatty tissue, less muscle tissue, and, therefore, a diminished need for body water and blood supply, which would dilute the alcohol.

8. In both genders, age-related increases in the ratio of body fat to lean muscle mass results in higher BACs for elders consuming the same amount of alcohol as they did when they were younger.

9. Certain signs and symptoms of alcohol consumption are similar to those of serious medical disorders unrelated to drinking.

Progress Test B (Chapters 3 & 4)

1. Persons with an alcoholic biological parent have about a 2.5-fold increased general risk for _____ _____.

2. Identical twins, even when they _____ _____, have a greater concordance than fraternal twins for drinking behavior and alcohol dependence.

3. Alcohol is a _____ at every level of brain functioning, affecting behavior and conscience.

4. As the body metabolizes alcohol, decreasing BAC, feelings of pleasure often change to _____ _____.

5. The most powerful predictor of alcohol use among young people is _____ _____.

6. Drinking one 12-ounce can of most beers represents an intake of _____ _____, the same as or greater than a 1.5-ounce serving of bourbon or gin.

7. Most alcohol is _____ through the small intestine and _____ by the liver.

8. A given volume of alcohol is higher in women than in men because women have smaller bodies, more _____ _____, and less muscle tissue.

9. A patient with a BAC of 0.15 g/dL, who _____ _____, will reach 0 BAC in about 10 hours.

Chapter 5 Diagnostic Criteria: Alcohol Abuse and Dependence

Diagnosis involves identifying and labeling specific disorders, e.g., alcohol abuse and alcohol dependence. Diagnostic criteria embody the consensus of researchers on which patterns of behavior and/or physiologic characteristics constitute distinguishing signs and symptoms. As new data become available, researchers revise criteria to improve their reliability, validity, and precision.

> Diagnosis involves identifying and labeling specific disorders, e.g., alcohol abuse and alcohol dependence.

Criteria sources currently used to diagnose alcohol abuse and alcohol dependence include:

1. *Diagnostic and Statistical Manual of Mental Disorders: DSM-IV,* published by the American Psychiatric Association (APA);[74] this standard work, which classifies all mental disorders (including substance abuse), is used mainly in the United States.

2. *International Classification of Diseases: ICD-10,* published by the World Health Organization (WHO);[76] this classification system for all causes of death and disability (including psychiatric orders) is used internationally.[77]

The DSM-IV and ICD-10 criteria are based on the most recent research findings and results of field trials. As the United States moves increasingly toward managed health care, third-party payers are requiring more standardized reporting of illnesses; they want to know what they are paying for and whether the standards are the same from program to program. Although clinical judgment will always play a role in diagnosing any illness, those clinicians using standardized diagnostic criteria will be in the best position to select appropriate treatments and to justify their selections to third-party payers.[77]

Demographics

Diagnostic criteria can be used in surveys, as well as for disorder assessment. In the NLAES, among the 42,862 persons interviewed, an estimated 7.4% met DSM-IV criteria for alcohol abuse or alcohol dependence during 1992; this figure represented approximately 13,760,000 Americans. In general, these disorders affected more men than women (11% vs. 4%) and more non-African Americans than African Americans (7.7% vs. 5.3%).[78]

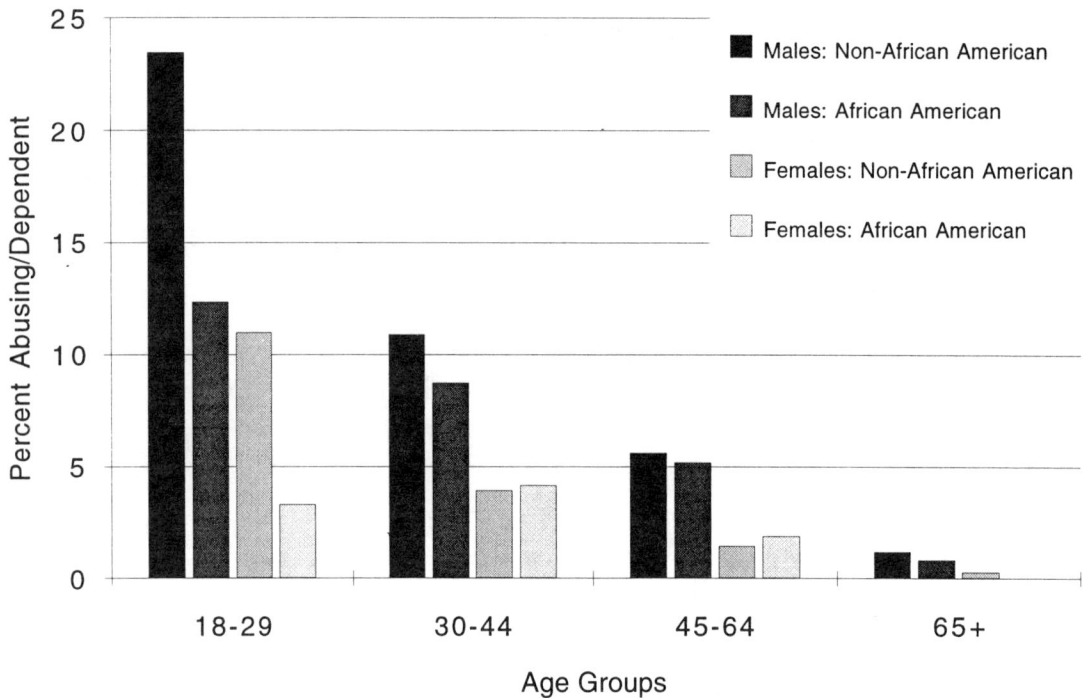

Fig. 8. Alcohol Abuse or Dependence Demographics, 1992, in the Contiguous United States and District of Columbia

Alcohol Abuse

Algorithm 1 gives the APA's DSM-IV diagnostic criteria for substance abuse, adapted to focus solely on alcohol.[74] No positive diagnosis can be made without first establishing a pattern of alcohol use. (*See Chapters 6 and 7 for preliminary testing and assessment.*)

Algorithm 1. Alcohol Abuse: DSM-IV Diagnostic Criteria			
Does patient exhibit:	**As manifested by ≥1 of following, occurring within a 12-month period:**	**And do:**	**If yes:**
A maladaptive pattern of alcohol use leading to clinically significant impairment or distress?	1. Recurrent alcohol use resulting in a failure to fulfill major role obligations at work, school, or home (e.g., repeated absences or poor work performance related to alcohol use; alcohol-related absences, suspensions, or expulsions from school; neglect of children or household) 2. Recurrent alcohol use in situations in which it is physically hazardous (e.g., driving an automobile or operating a machine when impaired by alcohol use) 3. Recurrent alcohol-related legal problems (e.g., arrests for alcohol-related disorderly conduct) 4. Continued alcohol use despite persistent or recurrent social or interpersonal problems caused or exacerbated by effects of the drug (e.g., arguments with spouse about consequences of intoxication; physical fights).	Results of the patient's physical examination, laboratory tests, and behavioral assessments support these criteria? (*See Chapters 6 & 7.*)	Consider diagnosis of alcohol abuse

Adapted, and reprinted with permission, from the Diagnostic and Statistical Manual of Mental Disorders, *4th edition. Copyright 1994 American Psychiatric Association.*

Rather than alcohol abuse, WHO uses the ICD-10 category called "harmful use," which requires that:

1. Alcohol use must have caused damage to the mental or physical health of the user, and
2. There is no concurrent diagnosis of alcohol dependence.[77]

Alcohol Dependence

The DSM-IV and ICD-10 diagnostic criteria for substance dependence (including alcohol) focus on an interrelated cluster of psychologic symptoms, physiologic signs, and behavioral indicators. Although the two standards are somewhat different, their similarities facilitate planning of treatment, collection of statistical data, and communication of research results worldwide. Table 11 compares the DSM-IV and ICD-10 criteria, showing their applications to alcohol dependence. As with alcohol abuse, in order to make a positive diagnosis, clinicians must first systematically determine if results of physical examinations, laboratory tests, and behavioral assessments support the diagnostic criteria.[74,77,79]

The risk for physiologic disorders and relapse is higher when a patient exhibits tolerance and/or withdrawal; therefore, the APA subdivides DSM-IV alcohol dependence diagnoses as follows:

1. <u>With</u> physiologic dependence—the ≥3 manifestations in Table 11 include either item 1 (tolerance) or item 2 (withdrawal)
2. <u>Without</u> physiologic dependence—the ≥3 manifestations in Table 11 do not include either item 1 or item 2.[74]

Table 11. Alcohol Dependence Comparison of DSM-IV* and ICD-10 Diagnostic Criteria		
FOCUS	**DSM-IV Symptoms:** a maladaptive pattern of alcohol use, leading to clinically significant impairment or distress as manifested by ≥3 of the following, occurring at any time in the same 12-month period:	**ICD-10 Symptoms:** patient has experienced or exhibited ≥3 of the following, at some time during the previous year:
Tolerance	1. A need for markedly increased amounts of alcohol to achieve intoxication or desired effect—or—a markedly diminished effect, from continued use of same amount of alcohol	1. Evidence of tolerance, such that increased doses are required to achieve effects originally produced by lower doses
Withdrawal	2. The characteristic alcohol withdrawal syndrome—or—ingestion of alcohol (or a closely related substance) to relieve or avoid withdrawal signs and symptoms	2. A physiologic withdrawal state when drinking has ceased or been reduced, as evidenced by the characteristic alcohol withdrawal syndrome—or—use of alcohol (or a closely related substance) to relieve or avoid withdrawal symptoms
Impaired Control	3. Frequent ingestion of alcohol in larger amounts or over longer periods than was intended 4. Persistent desire or unsuccessful efforts to cut down or control alcohol use	3. Difficulties in controlling drinking in terms of onset, termination, or levels of use 4. A strong desire or sense of compulsion to drink
Preoccupation With Drinking	5. Expenditure of a great deal of time on activities necessary to obtain or use alcohol, or to recover from its effects 6. Avoidance or reduction of important social, occupational, or recreational activities because of alcohol use	5. A great deal of time spent on activities necessary to obtain alcohol, to drink, or to recover from its effects—or—progressive neglect of alternative pleasures or interests in favor of drinking
Drinking Despite Problems	7. Continued drinking despite awareness of persistent or recurrent physiologic or mental disorders, most likely caused or exacerbated by the alcohol	6. Continued drinking despite clear evidence of overtly harmful physical or psychologic consequences

Adapted, and reprinted with permission, from the Diagnostic and Statistical Manual of Mental Disorders, 4th edition. Copyright 1994 American Psychiatric Association.

The potential alcohol dependence manifestations mentioned in Table 11 are further described below, except for alcohol withdrawal syndrome which is covered in Chapter 12.

Tolerance to Alcohol

Chronic drinkers often develop tolerance to alcohol. When the quantities of alcohol they usually drink no longer produce the desired effects, they must increase their intake. Tolerance is a useful clue to identifying patients who are starting to develop alcohol-related problems; e.g., younger patients who report they can "hold their liquor well."[80]

> *Joey's 17-year-old girlfriend, Sue, notices the bottle of whiskey on the floor of his car, parked facing a canal on the edge of the Everglades. "Don't you drink beer any more?" she asks. "Hell, no! Even when I drink a 6-pack, I don't feel anything," says Joey. "It takes half a bottle of this hard stuff to make me feel high." Joey takes a swig of whiskey and convinces Sue to do the same. About an hour and a half—and two thirds of a bottle—later, Joey starts the car and fumbles the shift into "drive." The car lurches forward into the canal. Joey struggles out through the open window on his side and manages to swim to shore. Shivering in the darkness, he looks at the water-filled car, and wishes he were strong enough to try to save Sue.*

Tolerance may be metabolic or functional. Metabolic tolerance occurs when the liver MEOS, activated after chronic drinking, accelerates alcohol metabolism; this reduces the duration and degree of intoxication.[80] Functional tolerance is believed to develop when, in response to acute or chronic alcohol exposure, conformation and functioning of cell-membrane molecules (i.e., lipids, proteins, and carbohydrates) are altered, and the number and/or functioning of certain neurotransmitter receptors (e.g., gamma-aminobutyric acid and norepinephrine) are altered.[2,81] (*See Chapter 8.*)

Functional tolerance is often seen in persons who drink on a daily basis; these chronic drinkers may exhibit few obvious signs of intoxication even at high BACs which, in others, would be incapacitating, even fatal.[80] Signs of chronic drinking can be more difficult to detect than, for example, those of binge drinking, in which behavioral pathology is often more pronounced.[13] (*See Student Binge Drinking, Chapter 2.*) Types of functional tolerance and factors influencing their development are:

1. Acute—during a single drinking session, the person's alcohol-induced impairment is greater soon after initial alcohol consumption than later in the drinking session, even if BAC is the same at both times.

2. Environment-dependent—over several drinking sessions, tolerance is accelerated if alcohol is always administered in the same

environment or is accompanied by the same cues; e.g., McCusker and Brown[82] found that males who drank socially performed eye-hand coordination tasks better (i.e., were more alcohol-tolerant) when drinking in a bar-like environment than when drinking in an office.

3. Learned—practicing a task while under the influence of alcohol can accelerate this phenomenon, called behaviorally augmented (i.e., learned) tolerance; e.g., Sdao-Jarvie[83] found that development of learned tolerance is accelerated when drinkers expect to receive money or another reward for a successful task performance, and Vogel-Sprott et al.[84] found that persons who had practiced an eye-hand coordination task after ingesting alcohol performed better than those who had practiced before drinking.[80]

One by one, the balls rise in perfect rhythm, as juggler Edward confidently tosses them, and the happy children watching him at the county fair are too far away to smell the liquor on his breath. Today, as on most other days, Edward performs his juggling act while intoxicated. Suddenly, coworker Pedro approaches him, saying: "My stomach ache is worse; I've got to go to the bathroom. Will you run the Ferris wheel, so I won't get in trouble?" Edward, who, when sober, had subbed for Pedro once before, starts up the passenger-filled Ferris wheel. Then, his mind blurs; he can't remember how and when to let passengers off. Ten minutes later, a passenger yells: "Hey, stop this thing! Enough is enough!"

Impaired Control

Drinkers are considered to have impaired control when they say they want to stop drinking but, even after repeated attempts, cannot do so. Impaired control also involves drinkers' inability to regulate the amount of alcohol consumed on a given occasion.[85]

Nancy swallows two Advil®, right after calling her boss to say she has a 102 °F fever and can't work today. She knows he probably doesn't believe her because she's had to call in sick a lot lately. Suddenly, she has to vomit and hurries to the bathroom; the Advil® go down the toilet as she flushes the foul vomitus. Later, as she lies on her bed, with her head still hurting unbearably, she vows, as she has so often before, to stop drinking. After about 10 hours, she awakens, feeling better, and gets up to watch television. The doorbell rings; it's her friend, Harry, holding a bottle of whiskey. As usual, Harry heads for the kitchen, where he mixes a couple of drinks, and, as usual, Nancy forgets her daily vow.

Preoccupation With Drinking

Alcohol-dependent persons are persistently preoccupied with drinking. They plan each waking moment around having a drink when they need it; when alcohol may be unavailable, they become almost frantic.[85]

Carlos half-fills his flask with the last of his vodka, then starts driving to the high school where he teaches algebra. In his classroom, he opens his briefcase to make sure the flask is there. He prays that the morning will pass quickly, so he can get a vodka boost at lunchtime. Who wouldn't drink, he thinks, if they had to spend their days disciplining a bunch of rowdies who didn't learn? Worst of all, it's Tuesday, and he has to tutor students all afternoon. When can he replenish his vodka supply? Carlos wipes the sweat from his forehead, as he anxiously tries to figure out how to get to the liquor store before tutoring begins. He decides the students can wait while he sneaks out for a half hour—his desperate need for a "vodka cushion" far outweighs starting the class on time.

Drinking Despite Problems

For alcohol-dependent persons, drinking has a far higher priority than other activities, and they continue to drink despite the many negative effects on their lives and those of others.

Ralph stands beside his car, staring at the teenager's body and the mangled bicycle on the street. The paramedic performing CPR on the boy is getting no response. A policeman leans toward Ralph, as if to smell his breath. "I'd like you to take a breath-alcohol test," he says. Ralph knows he can't refuse. Just last month, the same policeman had been at Ralph's house after his neighbors reported a loud argument with his wife. It seems like everything's going against him, he thinks. His boss has been complaining about his getting to work late and not doing his job properly. Even his kids don't seem to like him anymore. The paramedic looks at the policeman and says: "I did my best, but I couldn't revive him." Ralph staggers toward the paramedic and says: "He can't be dead; I never meant to kill anybody." The paramedic says, "What you meant didn't help this kid. He's gone."

Clinicians who treat patients such as those described above know that many alcohol-related problems can be prevented, if only the patients had been identified earlier. Most health care educational programs do not teach the techniques needed to identify alcohol misuse. The next two chapters in this course do.

Chapter Summary

1. Diagnostic criteria embody the consensus of researchers on which patterns of behavior and/or physiologic characteristics constitute distinguishing signs and symptoms.

2. Criteria sources currently used to diagnose alcohol abuse and alcohol dependence include the *Diagnostic and Statistical Manual of Mental Disorders: DSM-IV,* published by the American Psychiatric Association, and the *International Classification of Diseases: ICD-10,* published by the World Health Organization.

3. The DSM-IV diagnostic criteria for alcohol abuse include recurrent alcohol use in situations in which it is physically hazardous, and despite social or interpersonal problems caused or exacerbated by effects of the drug.

4. The DSM-IV and ICD-10 diagnostic criteria for alcohol dependence focus on an interrelated cluster of signs and symptoms, including tolerance, withdrawal, impaired control, preoccupation with drinking, and drinking despite problems.

5. No positive diagnosis of either alcohol abuse or dependence can be made without <u>first</u> establishing a pattern of alcohol use; the results of physical examinations, laboratory tests, and behavioral assessments must support the diagnostic criteria.

6. Tolerance may be metabolic (the liver MEOS accelerates alcohol metabolism) or functional (conformation and functioning of cell-membrane molecules are altered, and the number and/or functioning of certain neurotransmitter receptors are altered).

7. Types of functional tolerance are (1) acute, (2) environment-dependent, (3) learned.

8. Drinkers are considered to have impaired control when they say they want to stop drinking but, even after repeated attempts, cannot do so.

9. Alcohol-dependent persons continue to drink despite the many negative effects on their lives and those of others.

Chapter 6   Identifying Alcohol Misuse

Most clinical practices have many more patients who fall into the hazardous drinking or mild alcohol problem categories than who are already in the grip of alcohol abuse or alcohol dependence. (*For definitions of drinking categories, see Introduction.*) Unfortunately, clinicians often fail to identify alcohol misuse because they:

1. Believe such detection is not in the realm of their practices
2. Believe that, even if they do detect the problem, they cannot help the patient
3. Have not been trained to detect its less obvious indicators (e.g., patients may be asymptomatic in the early stages of alcohol misuse; others may avoid alcohol for several days prior to their appointments).

The challenge of identifying alcohol misuse is pointed up by a classic statement which Bissell[86] attributes to recovering alcoholics. Such patients, looking back on their early contacts with physicians, when diagnosis might have been made but was not, have often said: "I didn't volunteer the facts, and no one really asked."

> All clinicians should be highly sensitive to indicators of alcohol misuse.

All clinicians should be highly sensitive to indicators of alcohol misuse; e.g., a dental hygienist may learn of a symptom during conversation with a patient; a nurse may observe a sign while checking a patient's blood pressure. Such information, when passed on to dentists or physicians, promotes early identification of patients who are starting to misuse alcohol; it also promotes much-needed identification of chronic drinkers who have never sought or received help and/or those who have relapsed following treatment.

The tools used to identify alcohol misuse include patient histories, behavioral questionnaires, physical examinations, and laboratory tests. Algorithm 2 shows how these tools fit into an overall plan for identifying and treating alcohol misuse; use of the tools can be adapted or modified, depending on individual drinkers' needs and the specific responsibilities of clinics treating these patients.

Initial Steps

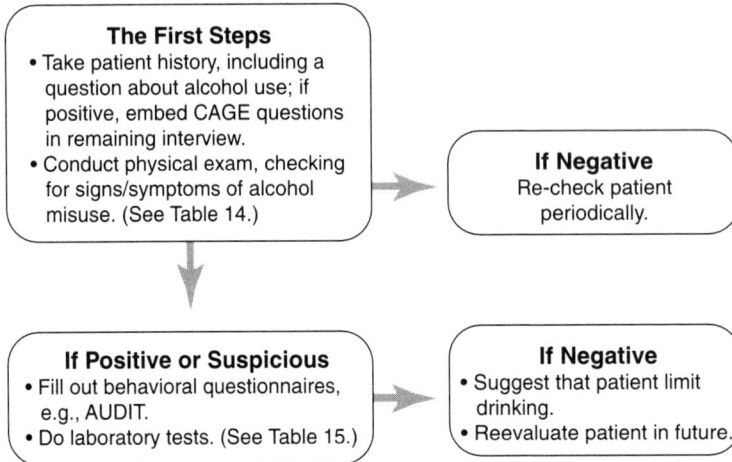

The First Steps
- Take patient history, including a question about alcohol use; if positive, embed CAGE questions in remaining interview.
- Conduct physical exam, checking for signs/symptoms of alcohol misuse. (See Table 14.)

If Negative
Re-check patient periodically.

If Positive or Suspicious
- Fill out behavioral questionnaires, e.g., AUDIT.
- Do laboratory tests. (See Table 15.)

If Negative
- Suggest that patient limit drinking.
- Reevaluate patient in future.

Follow-through Steps

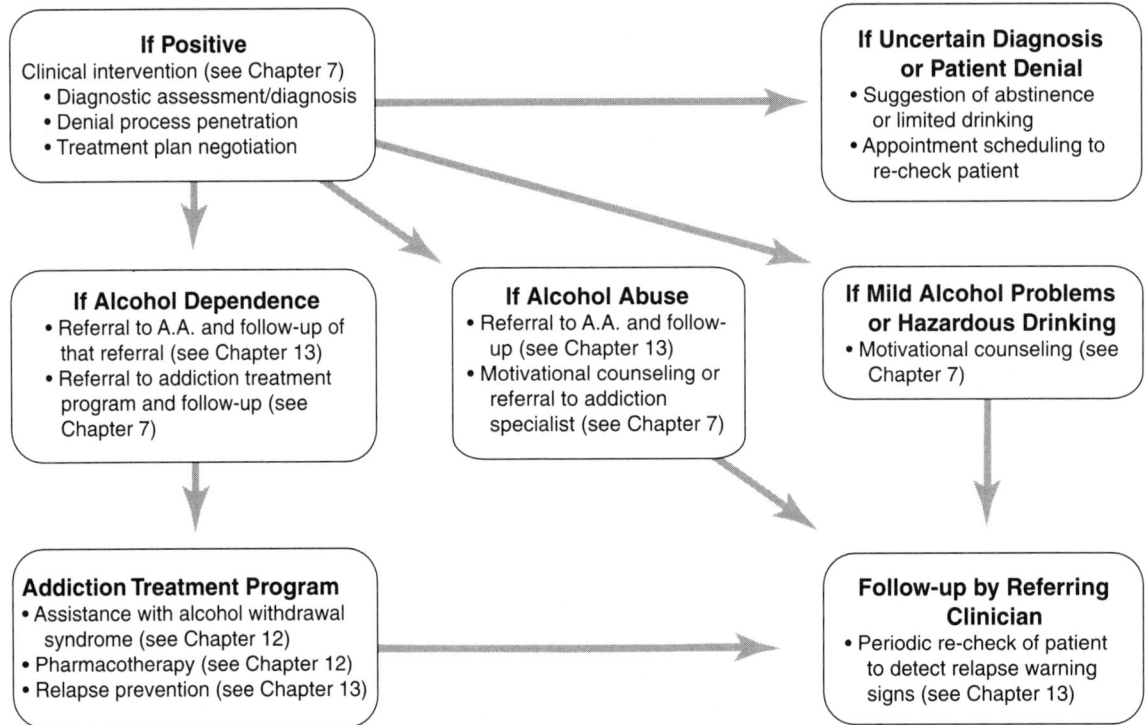

If Positive
Clinical intervention (see Chapter 7)
- Diagnostic assessment/diagnosis
- Denial process penetration
- Treatment plan negotiation

If Uncertain Diagnosis or Patient Denial
- Suggestion of abstinence or limited drinking
- Appointment scheduling to re-check patient

If Alcohol Dependence
- Referral to A.A. and follow-up of that referral (see Chapter 13)
- Referral to addiction treatment program and follow-up (see Chapter 7)

If Alcohol Abuse
- Referral to A.A. and follow-up (see Chapter 13)
- Motivational counseling or referral to addiction specialist (see Chapter 7)

If Mild Alcohol Problems or Hazardous Drinking
- Motivational counseling (see Chapter 7)

Addiction Treatment Program
- Assistance with alcohol withdrawal syndrome (see Chapter 12)
- Pharmacotherapy (see Chapter 12)
- Relapse prevention (see Chapter 13)

Follow-up by Referring Clinician
- Periodic re-check of patient to detect relapse warning signs (see Chapter 13)

Algorithm 2. Overview of Identifying, Diagnosing, and Treating Alcohol Misuse. Few clinicians will complete all these steps; however, most clinicians can assist at some point, then make referrals, and follow up on them.

Patient History

Health care workers responsible for taking patient histories should do so in private settings, where they can easily make eye contact. Patients who seem uncomfortable should be assured that their medical records are confidential.[87] (*See Observing Confidentiality, Chapter 7.*) Eliciting an accurate patient history requires tact, skill, patience, and understanding, and Table 12 shows some do's and don't's which could affect responses given by any patients, but, in particular, those who misuse alcohol.[86,87]

Table 12. Do's and Don't's of Taking Histories	
Do Try to: • Clarify the precise reason for patients' visits and acquire information to help you meet their needs	**And determine if patients are:** • Seeking relief from a symptom (e.g., anxiety, fatigue, abdominal pain, depression) • Trying to corroborate another physician's diagnosis • Looking for support of their belief that their lifestyles are not destructive.
Do be aware that: • Patients may not answer questions about alcohol use with absolute honesty	**And may be:** • Worried about having to stop drinking and endure alcohol withdrawal syndrome • Worried that health insurance won't pay bills for alcohol misuse treatment • Embarrassed about drinking and the problems it is creating • Continually lying to themselves, reinforcing the belief that they have no drinking problems.
Do offer only: • Factual medical information about alcohol misuse; judgmental comments alienate patients	**In case patients have:** • Wrestled psychologically, for a long time, with negative feelings about getting help; they have finally come to the clinic, believing they won't be judged, but will obtain some relief from their drinking problems.
Don't allow: • Staff questions or telephone calls to interrupt history taking	**Because:** • You may reverse already nervous patients' decisions to confide in you; e.g., they had planned to tell you about a drunk-driving accident or spouse abuse.
Don't leave: • Major inconsistencies in a health history unsettled	**Because:** • Your belief in patients' credibility may be undermined; e.g., first he says he drinks only on weekends while watching TV at home, and later says his wife gets upset when he goes out drinking with the guys a couple of nights a week.
Don't permit: • Patients to manipulate you to reject them or their behavior	**Because:** • This might justify patients' continued self-abuse; e.g., she thinks you've written her off as a "boozer," so she won't seek help.

History taking often begins with a few questions about aspects of patients' lives; many areas (e.g., relationships, work and/or school, health, behavior, finances, and law abidance) can be affected by alcohol misuse. Such questions not only provide basic psychosocial information, but allow development or renewal of clinician-patient relationships, before the more threatening questions, such as those about use of alcohol and other drugs, are asked.[88]

Clinicians should ask substance use questions in a consistent, matter-of-fact tone, while maintaining a supportive, nonjudgmental, and friendly (but not joking) attitude. Initial questions about use of alcohol and other drugs can be interspersed with those about smoking, caffeine intake, medication use, exercise, and sleep patterns; each response should be evaluated for denial, minimization, and rationalization.[79] Table 13 shows sample questions which can work the subject of alcohol use into patient histories. Clinicians taking this course should review the patient history questionnaires they currently use to see if they identify alcohol misuse.

Table 13. Alcohol and History Taking	
Make eye contact with patient and ask:	**If patient says "yes," then ask:**
Do you drink coffee? Tea?	About how many cups per day?
How about caffeinated soft drinks?	About how many per day?
Do you exercise regularly?	What is your exercise schedule like?
Have you had any trouble sleeping?	What do you think is causing this?
What over-the-counter medications do you take?	Can you think of any others?
Are you currently taking any prescription medications?	What kind? **Note:** if any are psychoactive like alcohol, clinicians should explore further: How long have you been taking the medication? Why are you taking it? How does it make you feel?
Do you smoke?	When did you start? How many cigarettes do you usually smoke per day?
Do you ever drink alcohol?	How often do you drink? About how many drinks? (*See comments below.*)
Do you have a family history of alcoholism?	Your father? Mother?
Have you ever used any street drugs?	What kind? How often?

If patients become nervous or hostile during questioning, clinician-interviewers should say: "I'm sorry if you feel uncomfortable about this, but please understand that we ask these questions of all our patients."[88] Patients may find it easy to report exactly how many cups of coffee they drink or how many cigarettes they smoke each day. However, when answering questions about alcohol use, they may shift to a less precise style ("I drink off and on," or "I take a few"). This clue signals a need for further investigation, not of the exact amounts patients consume, but of the effects drinking has on them.[86] Clinicians can obtain further information, without patients being aware of their suspicions, by casually embedding CAGE questions into the remainder of the interview. (*See CAGE in this chapter.*)

Physical Examination

Rarely do patients give alcohol misuse as the reason for their clinic visits. They are more likely to complain about a physiologic or mental disorder which, on the surface, appears wholly unrelated to drinking. Clinicians must then make the connection. Table 14 shows signs and symptoms of alcohol misuse which clinicians may notice during a physical examination.[89,90,91]

Table 14. Alcohol-related Physical Examination	
When examining:	**Among other possibilities, check for:**
Skin	• Erythema of face/palms • Dilated venules • Beard folliculitis • Psoriasis • Rosacea and rhinophyma • Seborrheic dermatitis • Florid vascular spiders
Eyes	• Arcus senilis • Nystagmus
Mouth	• Coated tongue • Poor oral hygiene • Advanced periodontitis • Angular cheilitis • Glossitis • Ulcerations • Xerostomia • Dental attrition secondary to bruxism • Increased DMF rate (decayed/missing/filled teeth)
Cardiovascular function	• Hypertension • Palpitations • Tachycardia • Atrial fibrillation
Respiratory function	• Upper respiratory infections, bronchitis, pneumonia (ask for history, too)
Musculoskeletal appearance	• Gout • Myopathy of the shoulder • Dupuytren's contracture
When asking about:	**Among other possibilities, check for:**
Digestive tract disorders	• Morning nausea/vomiting • Gastroesophageal reflux • Vomiting of blood • Dysphagia • Recurrent diarrhea • Anorexia • Abdominal/stomach pain
Reproductive disorders	• Impotence • Irregular menstruation
Neurologic/mental disorders	• Peripheral neuropathy • Insomnia • Anxiety • Suicidal thoughts • Amnesia • Tremor • Seizure • Depression

General signs of chronic alcohol misuse include puffiness of the face and eyelids, parotid gland swelling, hand tremor, unexplained cuts and bruises, and the odor of alcohol on the breath. Patients who drink and smoke might have cigarette burns, tobacco stains, hoarseness, or heavy coughs. Diagnosis and treatment of serious alcohol-related disorders are discussed in Chapters 9 and 10. As shown in Algorithm 2, if patient histories and physical examinations are negative for alcohol misuse, clinicians should simply re-check patients periodically. However, if the results are positive or suspicious, clinicians should conduct further screening, as discussed below.

Behavioral Questionnaires

Behavioral questionnaires (also called "screening instruments") are used to determine the <u>existence</u> of alcohol misuse; they do not measure the <u>extent</u> of alcohol-related problems or establish a definitive diagnosis. They are designed to detect:

1. Loss of control over drinking, as perceived by the patient and others
2. Continued drinking despite the problems it creates
3. Evidence of alcohol tolerance and alcohol withdrawal syndrome.[13]

Because these questionnaires are highly sensitive, they will detect most alcohol misuse. However, they have <u>lower specificity</u>, which means they might give false-positive results for persons who drink alcohol, but do not misuse it. To minimize possible adverse consequences (e.g., denial of health insurance), positive results should be followed up with a diagnostic assessment.[2] (*See Chapter 7.*)

Clinicians can ask: "Do you feel your drinking is causing any problems?"

To motivate patients to participate in this screening, clinicians can ask: "Do you feel your drinking is causing any problems?" Patients may answer: "Perhaps," or "I'm not sure; how can I find out?" Such patients are usually willing to answer the behavioral questions discussed below. If patients decline to participate, clinicians should urge them to limit their drinking and schedule a follow-up appointment.

The brief CAGE behavioral questionnaire is usually incorporated into conversations with patients. (*See page 69.*) Longer questionnaires are administered as face-to-face interviews, or as paper-and-pencil or self-guided computerized tests.[2] Their use with adolescents is controversial; some researchers believe a skilled interviewer elicits more valid information than a questionnaire. In either case, and for any age group, accurate responses depend on patients' trust in those administering the questionnaires.[92]

CAGE

C	Have you ever felt you ought to **C**ut down on your drinking?
A	Have people **A**nnoyed you by criticizing your drinking?
G	Have you ever felt bad or **G**uilty about your drinking?
E	Have you ever had a drink first thing in the morning (**E**ye opener) to steady your nerves or get rid of a hangover?

Questions reprinted with permission. Ewing JA. Detecting alcoholism: the CAGE questionnaire. *Journal of the American Medical Association.* 1984;252(14):1905-1907.

CAGE, because of its brevity, is very useful in clinical practices, trauma centers, and hospitals. Two or more positive responses indicate "possible" alcohol abuse or dependence; <u>even one</u> positive answer means the patient warrants further assessment. This test evaluates lifetime, <u>not</u> current, drinking; it does not apply to episodes of acute alcohol use or measure levels of consumption. Clinicians should not ask CAGE questions in a formal, exam-like style; they should embed them in conversations during history taking or physical examinations.

> *Did you see the story on the news about the quarterback who was arrested for drunk driving? That's the third time in 6 months. You'd think he'd have enough sense to at least cut down on his drinking.* **Have you ever felt you ought to cut down on your drinking?** *Seems one of his friends tried to get him to stop, and the quarterback punched him out.* **Have people annoyed you by criticizing your drinking?** *Can you imagine how the quarterback would have felt had he hurt or killed someone while he was driving drunk?* **Have you ever felt bad or guilty about your drinking?** *I heard that this guy has to have a drink as soon as he gets out of bed, just so he can put his clothes on.* **Have you ever had a drink first thing in the morning—an eye opener—to steady your nerves or get rid of a hangover?**

SMAST

The original 25-question Michigan Alcoholism Screening Test (MAST), developed by Selzer in 1971, set the stage for shorter variants; one these is SMAST, which evaluates lifetime <u>and</u> current drinking. To help identify patients in the <u>early</u> stages of problem drinking, Fleming[93] suggests that clinicians add the following questions when using CAGE and MAST (or SMAST):

1. To determine frequency: How many days per week do you drink?
2. To determine quantity: On a day when you drink alcohol, how many drinks do you have?
3. To determine binge drinking: On how many occasions in the last month did you have more than five drinks?[94]

SMAST has 13 questions, scored as follows: 0-1=nonalcoholic; 2=possibly alcoholic; ≥3 or "yes" to questions 6, 10, or 11=alcoholic.

Short Michigan Alcoholism Screening Test (SMAST)	
Question	Answer = Points
1. Do you feel you are a "normal" drinker? (By normal, we mean you drink less than or as much as most other people.)	No = 1
2. Does your wife, husband, a parent, or other near relative ever worry or complain about your drinking?	Yes = 1
3. Do you ever feel guilty about your drinking?	Yes = 1
4. Do friends or relatives think you are a "normal" drinker?	No = 1
5. Are you able to stop drinking when you want to?	No = 1
6. Have you ever attended a meeting of Alcoholics Anonymous?	Yes = 1
7. Has drinking ever created problems between you and your wife, husband, a parent, or other near relative?	Yes = 1
8. Have you ever gotten into trouble at work because of your drinking?	Yes = 1
9. Have you ever neglected your obligations, your family, or your work for 2 or more days in a row because you were drinking?	Yes = 1
10. Have you ever gone to anyone for help about your drinking?	Yes = 1
11. Have you ever been in a hospital because of drinking?	Yes = 1
12. Have you ever been arrested for drunken driving, driving while intoxicated, or driving under the influence of alcoholic beverages?	Yes = 1
13. Have you ever been arrested, even for a few hours, because of drunken behavior?	Yes = 1
TOTAL SCORE:	

Questions reprinted with permission from Selzer ML, Vinokur A, Van Rooijen L. A self-administered Short Michigan Alcoholism Screening Test (SMAST). *Journal of Studies on Alcohol.* 1975;36(1):117-126.

AUDIT

The AUDIT 10-item questionnaire, which assesses the extent of drinking and resultant problems during the preceding 12 months, is specifically designed to screen for alcohol misuse at early stages. A score of ≥8 may indicate the need for a more in-depth assessment.[95]

California law requires physicians to report to local health departments all patients >14 years old who, during the preceding 3 years, had episodes of unconsciousness or marked confusion resulting from any condition which may cause relapses (e.g., diabetes mellitus or alcohol-induced amnesia). AUDIT question no. 8 could elicit answers requiring such reporting.[96] Therefore, in California and any other states with this law, Kitchens[97] recommends that physicians trying to determine whether patients are at-risk drinkers use CAGE, supplemented by the first three AUDIT questions.

Alcohol Use Disorders Identification Test (AUDIT)						
Circle the number that comes closest to your actions <u>during the past year</u>						
1. How often do you have a drink containing alcohol?	• Never • Monthly or less • 2-4 times a month • 2-3 times a week • 4 or more times a week	0 1 2 3 4	6. How often have you needed a first drink in the morning to get yourself going after an episode of acute alcohol use?	• Never • Less than monthly • Monthly • Weekly • Daily or almost daily	0 1 2 3 4
2. How many drinks containing alcohol do you have on a typical day when you are drinking?	• 1 or 2 • 3 or 4 • 5 or 6 • 7 to 9 • 10 or more	0 1 2 3 4	7. How often have you had a feeling of guilt or remorse after drinking?	• Never • Less than monthly • Monthly • Weekly • Daily or almost daily	0 1 2 3 4
3. How often do you have 6 or more drinks on 1 occasion?	• Never • Less than monthly • Monthly • Weekly • Daily or almost daily	0 1 2 3 4	8. How often have you been unable to remember what happened the night before because you had been drinking?	• Never • Less than monthly • Monthly • Weekly • Daily or almost daily	0 1 2 3 4
4. How often have you found that you were not able to stop drinking once you had started?	• Never • Less than monthly • Monthly • Weekly • Daily or almost daily	0 1 2 3 4	9. Have you or someone else been injured as a result of your drinking?	• Never • Less than monthly • Monthly • Weekly • Daily or almost daily	0 1 2 3 4
5. How often have you failed to do what was normally expected from you because of drinking?	• Never • Less than monthly • Monthly • Weekly • Daily or almost daily	0 1 2 3 4	10. Has a relative, friend, or doctor or other health worker been concerned about your drinking or suggested you cut down?	• Never • Less than monthly • Monthly • Weekly • Daily or almost daily	0 1 2 3 4
				SUM OF ITEM SCORES:	

Source: Developed by the World Health Organization, AMETHYST Project, 1987.

Questionnaires for Special Groups

For the most part, the standard behavioral questionnaires were developed for use with men. They can be used for women and adolescents, but the sensitivity of their answers is increased if questionnaires developed for these particular groups are used.[91]

The TWEAK test is designed specifically to ascertain alcohol misuse by women. Blume[24] suggests that, to recognize the frequency of multiple drug use, the "E" question might be better worded: "Have you ever needed a drink, or medication of some kind, first thing in the morning?" The "A" question poses the same challenge for California physicians as does AUDIT question 8. On TWEAK's 7-point scale, a total score of 3 or more points indicates that a woman may well have an alcohol abuse or alcohol dependence problem.[98]

Do you drink alcoholic beverages? If so, please take our TWEAK test.	Answer	Points
Tolerance: How many drinks does it take to make you feel high?	Record number of drinks: ____ (if 2 or more, enter 2 at right)	____
Worry: Have close friends or relatives worried or complained about your drinking in the past year?	If Yes, enter 2 at right	____
Eye opener: Do you sometimes take a drink in the morning when you first get up?	If Yes, enter 1 at right	____
Amnesia (blackouts): Has a friend or family member ever told you about things you said or did while you were drinking that you could not remember?	If Yes, enter 1 at right	____
Do you sometimes feel the need to Cut down on your drinking? (C stands for the K)	If Yes, enter 1 at right	____
	TOTAL SCORE:	

Source: Russell M., Martier SS, Sokol RJ, et al. Screening for pregnancy risk-drinking: TWEAK-ing the tests. Abstract. *Alcoholism: Clinical and Experimental Research.* 1991;15(2):368.

Descriptions of several behavioral questionnaires for adolescents appear in *Assessing Drug Abuse Among Adolescents and Adults: Standardized Instruments,* NIH Publication No. 94-3757, available from the National Clearinghouse for Alcohol and Drug Information (NCADI): 1-800-729-6686 or 1-301-468-2600.

If the results of history taking, the physical examination, and behavioral questionnaires raise suspicions of alcohol misuse by any patient, clinicians should consider further screening, involving biological state markers.

Biological State Markers

Laboratory-derived signs of excessive and harmful alcohol consumption can be divided into two main groups: trait markers and state markers. Genetic <u>trait</u> markers, which may someday be used to identify people susceptible to alcohol dependence, were discussed in Chapter 3. (*See Table 7.*) Biological <u>state</u> markers, which can detect recent or chronic drinking, are abnormal or elevated values of certain molecules (e.g., alcohol) in blood, breath, or urine; a state marker detecting episodes of heavy drinking involves mean corpuscular volume. (*See Table 15.*)[13,99,100]

Table 15. Biological State Markers	
To identify:	Test for:
Recent drinking	Alcohol, acetate, and/or methanol in blood
	Alcohol in breath
	5-hydroxytryptophol (5-HTOL) in urine
Chronic drinking	Gamma-glutamyl transferase (GGT) in blood serum
Heavy drinking	Increased mean corpuscular volume (MCV)

Alcohol in Blood and Breath

Blood samples give specific BAC; but, in some settings, breath samples are more easily obtained. The breath-alcohol concentration (BrAC) in end-expiratory breath accurately reflects the pulmonary BAC (end-expiratory breath is a full exhalation's last one third, in which alcohol has reached a concentration "plateau"). Using breath-alcohol analyzers (e.g., the Breathalyzer®) as a field laboratory, police collect these specimens. This noninvasive measurement of BrAC at the site of a motor vehicle crash allows police to make immediate decisions about their further actions.[101]

Gamma-glutamyl Transferase

Currently, the enzyme gamma-glutamyl transferase (GGT) is the individual state marker most often employed to detect chronic alcohol misuse, which causes GGT to be released from the liver into the bloodstream.[99] GGT, which has normal values of <40 I.U./L of blood serum,[91] is elevated in about two thirds of alcoholic-dependent persons.[13] When GGT exceeds 60 I.U./L of blood serum, the probability that a patient has been consuming >6 drinks per day over a period of weeks increases from 20% to 50%. However, clinicians must eliminate the possibility of such nonalcoholic causes of elevated GGT as: severe trauma; certain heart and kidney diseases; all types of liver diseases; barbiturates and medications used to treat epilepsy and blood-clotting disorders; obesity/dietary factors (patient is 30% overweight or has elevated blood fat levels).[99]

Mean Corpuscular Volume

Mean corpuscular volume (MCV), or macrocytosis, correlates positively with the duration of a drinking episode and the amount of alcohol consumed. Seppä[102] found that the incidence of macrocytosis among patients in general practice was 2.4%; of those patients with macrocytosis, 80.2% of the men and 34.1% of the women had misused alcohol. Before suspecting alcohol abuse or dependence, clinicians must exclude other causes of increased MCV, such as deficiencies of nutrients (e.g., vitamin B_{12} and folate), liver disease, reticulocytosis, antiepileptic drugs, increased age, smoking, and menopause.[99]

Other State Markers

Elevated levels of triglycerides, alkaline phosphatase, bilirubin, and uric acid can indicate liver damage and, perhaps, heavy drinking. Elevated levels of carbohydrate-deficient transferrin (CDT) occur in about 80% of people who drink heavily for ≥1 week; this marker is being intensively studied because it is highly specific for liver disease caused by consumption of large quantities of alcohol.[13]

Researchers are testing combinations of markers in an effort to achieve better sensitivity and specificity in identifying recent and chronic drinking. Currently, many patients who drink heavily do not have abnormal test results, and many patients with abnormal test results are not alcohol-dependent.[13] In the meantime, clinicians can use findings of elevated levels of single markers to motivate patients to cut down their drinking.[99]

Clinicians use laboratory tests to corroborate suspicions generated by results of patient histories, physical examinations, and behavioral questionnaires. Chapter 7 discusses diagnostic assessments; if patients refuse to participate in these assessments, clinicians should immediately schedule another appointment, and urge the patients to abstain from, or, at least, limit their drinking.

Chapter Summary

1. All clinicians should be highly sensitive to indicators of alcohol misuse; such information promotes <u>early</u> identification of patients who are starting to misuse alcohol and <u>much-needed</u> identification of chronic drinkers.

2. Tools used to identify alcohol misuse include patient histories, behavioral questionnaires, physical examinations, and laboratory tests.

3. Patients who seem uncomfortable during history taking should be assured that their medical records are confidential.

4. Eliciting an accurate history involving alcohol use requires tact, skill, patience, and understanding.

5. Clinician-interviewers should ask substance use questions in a consistent, matter-of-fact tone, while maintaining a supportive, nonjudgmental, and friendly attitude.

6. General signs of chronic alcohol misuse include puffiness of the face and eyelids, parotid gland swelling, hand tremor, unexplained cuts and bruises, and the odor of alcohol on the breath.

7. Behavioral questionnaires are used to determine the <u>existence</u> of alcohol misuse; they do not measure the <u>extent</u> of alcohol-related problems or establish a definitive diagnosis.

8. Behavioral questionnaires determining alcohol misuse include:
    1. CAGE—evaluates lifetime, <u>not</u> current, drinking
    2. SMAST—evaluates lifetime <u>and</u> current drinking
    3. AUDIT—assesses the extent of drinking and resultant problems during the preceding 12 months
    4. TWEAK—specifically ascertains alcohol misuse by women.

9. Biological state markers used detect recent or chronic drinking are abnormal or elevated values of certain molecules in blood, breath, or urine; a state marker used to detect episodes of heavy drinking involves mean corpuscular volume.

Progress Test C (Chapters 5 & 6)

1. DSM-IV, a standard for classifying mental disorders, is used mainly in the
    _____ _____; ICD-10, a standard for classifying all causes of
    death and disability, is used _____.

2. Approximately 13,760,000 Americans met DSM-IV criteria for alcohol
    _____ or _____ during 1992.

3. Alcohol _____ is a useful clue to identifying patients who are
    starting to develop alcohol-related problems.

4. Drinkers with _____ _____ cannot stop drinking, even
    after repeated attempts to do so.

5. Clinicians should review the _____ _____
    questionnaires they currently use to see if they identify alcohol misuse.

6. Patients rarely give _____ _____ as the reason for their
    clinical visits.

7. General signs of chronic alcohol misuse include eyelid puffiness,
    _____ _____ swelling, hand tremor, and unexplained cuts and
    bruises.

8. Because of its brevity, the behavioral questionnaire _____ is very useful in
    clinical practices, trauma centers, and hospitals.

9. The individual state marker most often employed to detect chronic alcohol
    misuse is the enzyme _____.

Chapter 7   Clinical Intervention

Intervention, a planned interaction with patients who misuse alcohol, involves:

1. <u>Diagnosing</u> the extent of patients' alcohol misuse (e.g., mild alcohol problems, alcohol abuse, or alcohol dependence)
2. <u>Assisting</u> patients to overcome denial; timing and context are important (e.g., during clinical visits for treatment of a severe alcohol-related disorder, sober patients are more likely to realize their drinking is affecting their health)
3. <u>Motivating</u> patients to abstain from, or reduce their consumption of, alcohol; clinicians' attitudes can make a difference (e.g., cooperative alliances change behavior more effectively than authoritarian stances)
4. <u>Negotiating</u> a treatment plan; a realistic plan tailors treatment to available services and patients' characteristics (e.g., patients' learning styles and motivational levels must be considered).[103,104]

Several studies have shown that even brief clinical interventions can reduce patient drinking.[1] Benzer and Winslow[105] suggest that: "The only <u>unsuccessful</u> intervention is one that is not done." However, practical problems for clinicians include:

1. Little or no medical school training in such ancillary skills as effective listening and patient negotiation
2. Failure to monitor patient compliance with referrals to addiction specialists (patients often do not follow through unless they are monitored).[104]

Making a Diagnosis

When results of questionnaires or tests in Chapter 6 are positive, clinicians should urge patients to be further evaluated by clinicians trained to use and interpret diagnostic questionnaires (or psychometric instruments). The goals of these assessments are: to obtain a <u>diagnosis</u>, assess the <u>severity</u> of patients' alcohol misuse, and determine patients' potential for rehabilitation. Before authorizing addiction treatment, many third-party payers require that these three goals be achieved.[106]

Before administering diagnostic questionnaires, clinicians must have clear answers to the following:

1. What are the patients' typical and maximum daily consumptions of alcohol, including:
   a. What types of alcoholic beverages are involved?
   b. When are the drinks consumed (e.g., between or with meals)? (*Answering these questions requires that an agreement be reached on what constitutes a drink—see Table 8.*)
2. Do the patients have a history of binge drinking?
3. Do the patients have histories of drinking before potentially dangerous activities (e.g., boating or driving an automobile)?
4. What are the patients' perceptions of their drinking?
   a. Do they feel they drink too much, and, if so, why?
   b. Are they interested in drinking less?
   c. Have they ever tried to change their drinking habits?[4]

Most patients view assessment questionnaires as a way to improve self-knowledge; others initially resist being interviewed, but, once the diagnostic clinician demonstrates a conversational (rather than checklist) style of questioning, they generally respond. Frequent breaks in questioning also increase the likelihood of responses.[106]

When assessment interviews do not lead to certain diagnoses, clinicians should consider gathering more diagnostic data by convening a family meeting at the clinic; however, the patient must agree to and be present at the meeting.[91] Such a meeting might also involve an employer, friend, or clergy person.

> *David says: "This meeting is a waste of time! I don't have a drinking problem." The diagnostic clinician says: "Mr. Rhodes, here, says you've missed work six times this month, and he's worried he might have to let you go." "I've had the flu and can't seem to shake it," says David. "But Mr. Rhodes says you were absent as much last month and the month before, and your buddy, Bill, here, says he's really concerned that you insisted on driving home drunk last Saturday night," says the clinician. "These people really care about you. Are you willing to take another look at your drinking habits?"*

Another way to learn more about the patient is to make the suggestion that the patient abstain from alcohol for 1 month (or limit alcohol use to 2 drinks per day for 2 months) and see what happens.

Clinicians can also learn from "watchful waiting," not making any recommendations, but carefully monitoring patients during regular follow-up appointments.[91]

Penetrating the Denial Process

Patients who misuse alcohol always find excuses for their drinking. Though they may feel guilty about gradually destroying their lives and health, they practice self-deception, lying to themselves to rationalize their drinking.

> *As she prepares supper, Patsy thinks about her husband, Matthew, and the years of misery she has endured because of his drinking. During the past week, he has attended Alcoholics Anonymous meetings 4 times, and has abstained from alcohol. She is really proud of him. The phone rings, interrupting Patsy's thoughts of a happier future. It's Matthew. "Honey, I had a really rotten day at the office, so I'm going to stop at Harry's Bar for just one quick drink before coming home. Don't worry. It's no big deal, just one drink, and I deserve it after all of today's problems." Patsy remembers these words at midnight, when Matthew comes home drunk and punches her in the face because she didn't keep his supper warm.*

Clinicians face a challenge when they must give patients diagnoses of alcohol abuse or dependence. Before patients can accept such diagnoses, they must first overcome their denial of alcohol misuse, realize the consequences of their drinking habits, and decide to accept help. To aid patients in achieving these goals, clinicians can use a type of encouragement called benevolent coercion; this involves demonstrating genuine concern for patients by expressing feelings such as sadness, embarrassment, or fearfulness (never anger or frustration). They must also:

1. Carefully explain clinical findings, using data collected from the history, physical examination, laboratory studies, and assessments.
2. Make sure patients understand both the findings and the fact that they indicate alcohol misuse.
3. Explain to patients that any current disorders will only worsen with continued alcohol misuse.[105]

Patients may respond to diagnoses of alcohol abuse or dependence with agitation, anger, sulking, or silence. Clinicians must remain calm, ready for whatever reactions are provoked: "I know this news upsets you." They must also be prepared to answer questions about treatment options, health coverage, and other issues.[105,107]

Because denial is difficult to overcome, clinicians should assure patients of continued access to care no matter what decisions they make about changing their drinking habits. Future visits for treatment of other medical disorders will serve as opportunities for clinicians to readdress issues of alcohol misuse, further educating the patients and discussing their diagnoses.[90]

Motivating Patients

Patients are ultimately responsible for changing their behavior, and their readiness to make such changes varies greatly. Once patients overcome denial, clinicians can motivate them to change their drinking habits by:

1. Urging them to attend a local A.A. meeting (*See Chapter 13.*)
2. Referring them to a psychosocial therapist for cognitive-behavioral therapy (*See Chapter 13.*) **Note**: to <u>avoid</u> violating confidentiality laws, see Consent Form in this chapter.
3. Asking them to:
    a. Prepare a list of the benefits of drinking versus the risks of drinking; then, think of other ways to achieve the same benefits
    b. Identify psychologic and social influences associated with their drinking and methods of dealing with them.[108]
4. Suggesting—if abstinence is <u>not</u> an option—they try moderate drinking.

Moderate Drinking

Clinicians often disagree on whether the goal of addiction treatment should be abstinence or moderate drinking. Some clinicians believe the option of moderate drinking can be used to motivate patients diagnosed with alcohol abuse (<u>not</u> alcohol dependence), provided they do not have physiologic or mental disorders contraindicating <u>any</u> alcohol consumption. (The U.S. Department of Agriculture defines moderate drinking as a maximum of 2 drinks per day for males; 1 drink per day for females).[109]

> The U.S. Department of Agriculture defines moderate drinking as a maximum of 2 drinks per day for males; 1 drink per day for females.

The first step in a moderate drinking program is a patient-clinician agreement on the patient's specific drinking goal and techniques to be used to achieve that goal, e.g., keeping a daily drinking diary, interspersing nonalcoholic beverages, diluting drinks, and slowing the rate of drinking.[4]

Sanchez-Craig and Lei[110] recommend that, before attempting moderate drinking, patients abstain from alcohol for 3 weeks to prove to themselves that they can control their drinking.[2] Clinicians monitoring patient moderate drinking programs should:

1. Call the patients after 2 weeks to determine if they are remaining abstinent or keeping to the agreed-upon alcohol limit.
2. See the patients once a month to support positive behavioral changes.[111]
3. Convince the patients to attend local self-help groups concentrating on moderate drinking, if such groups are available (most focus on abstinence).[4]

Patients who try moderate drinking, but fail to control their consumption, may be more open to abstinence as a treatment goal.[4]

Negotiating a Treatment Plan

Once patients are motivated to change their drinking habits, clinicians can facilitate their entering treatment by:

1. Offering hope for rehabilitation: "In my experience, patients like you have a high success rate."
2. Explaining possible courses of treatment and suggesting one, then letting patients share in planning it: "We'll work together on this."[107]

Because of the severity of their disorders, alcohol-dependent patients need care by addiction specialists; however, these patients often fail to follow up on referrals for reasons including fear of stigmatization, lack of insurance coverage, and/or anxiety about undergoing withdrawal. To provide for such patients, some clinics have on-staff addiction specialists; others ask specialists to consult with the patients at the clinics. However, most patients are referred to one of the types of settings described in Table 16.[112]

In recent years, inpatient treatment programs have undergone two major changes:

1. The length of stay in many programs has decreased dramatically because of increased emphasis on outpatient interventions and cost pressures from the insurance industry.
2. The patient population contains increasing numbers of multiple substance abusers; consequently, many programs now focus on alcohol and other drug (AOD) dependence rather than on alcohol dependence alone.[112]

Referring clinicians should advise patients to obtain a second opinion from the specialists. They should also arrange for feedback from the specialists so they can participate in treatment planning and, during subsequent visits, support patients' specific programs.[111]

| Table 16. Alcohol Addiction Treatment Settings ||
Types	Characteristics
Inpatient: intensive, highly structured care	• Medical disorder management • Psychosocial evaluation • Individual counseling to develop and implement a treatment plan • Personalized therapy for special problems or needs • Group therapy, several hours daily, once patient is sober • Education, e.g., health consequences of drinking, effects on family • 24-hour monitoring; expensive
Outpatient: intensive care	• Patients can practice relapse prevention and management skills in a highly structured setting (*See Chapter 13.*) • Evening programs for employed patients • Patients can maintain their roles of employee, spouse, and/or parent while receiving intensive treatment • Range of treatment time: from 3 hrs a day, several days a week, to 8 hrs a day, 7 days a week; significantly less expensive than inpatient care
Outpatient: regular care	• Participation in A.A. meetings (*See Chapter 13.*) • Weekly group therapy sessions • Regular individual counseling sessions • Used as primary treatment, or as extended aftercare following completion of either of the above types • Duration: generally 1 year, but number of treatment sessions relates to patient's progress and third-party payer coverage; less expensive than the above types

If alcohol-dependent patients refuse or lack financial resources to see addiction specialists, referring clinicians should:

1. Provide the patients with information about local A.A. meetings and urge them to attend.
2. Ask recovering, alcohol-dependent patients in their practices if they would be willing to meet with the newly diagnosed patients to discuss methods they have been using to change their own drinking habits.[111] **Note**: to <u>avoid</u> violating confidentiality laws, see Consent Form in this chapter.

Making a Referral List

All offices and clinics should have lists of current referral telephone numbers for sources of treatment of alcohol misuse and related disorders. Clinicians can identify public and private resources in their communities by:

1. Asking colleagues for names of treatment programs or individual providers
2. Contacting mental health centers or hospitals

3. Calling state agencies (*See National Prevention Network in Appendix A for a particular state's listing.*)
4. Calling the Center for Substance Abuse Treatment (CSAT) hot line: 1-800-662-HELP.[111]

The "Local Resources Form" in Appendix C, can be copied, filled in, and posted in reception areas, examining rooms, or nursing stations.[111]

Observing Confidentiality Laws

Confidentiality allows patients to determine when and to whom information about their diagnoses and treatment may be disclosed. Federal regulations guarantee confidentiality of information about all persons applying for or receiving services for alcohol and other drug (AOD) abuse problems; services may include screening, assessment, diagnosis, referral, individual or group counseling, or treatment. The regulations—Title 42, Part 2, Code of Federal Regulations (CFR)—are part of the Public Health Service Act, Title 42, Section 290dd-3, CFR.[113]

> Private practitioners should treat their AOD records as if the federal regulations applied to them.

The AOD confidentiality laws apply to federally assisted programs (those directly funded, operated, and/or licensed by the federal government; certified for Medicaid reimbursement; receiving federal block grant funds through a state or local government; exempt from paying federal taxes). State licensing authorities also abide by the federal regulations; for safety's sake, private practitioners should treat their AOD records as if the federal regulations applied to them.

Clinicians violate the federal regulations when they disclose patients' records, testify about patients' treatment, confirm that patients are being examined, interviewed, or treated, and/or pass on anecdotal material from which patients' identities may be inferred. Violators of the regulations are subject to a criminal penalty (up to $500 for the first offense; up to $5,000 for each subsequent offense). Violators jeopardize their licenses or certifications, and patients may sue violators for unauthorized disclosure.[113]

Consent Form

Anyone having information identifying participants in, or applicants for, AOD treatment may not disclose it without written patient consent or that of an authorized representative when necessary. Patients are generally given a written referral to an addiction specialist; however, if clinicians decide to make any referral calls themselves, even with patients present, they must first obtain patients' written consent on a form meeting federal regulations (<u>not</u> a general medical release form); the information which <u>must</u> be included is shown below.[113]

Consent Form for the Release of Confidential AOD Abuse Information

I, _____authorize
(Name of patient)

_____
(Name or general designation of program making disclosure)

to disclose to _____

the following information: _____
(Nature of the information, as limited as possible)

_____

_____

The purpose of the disclosure authorized herein is to _____

_____
(Disclosure purpose, as specific as possible)

I understand that my records are protected under the federal regulations governing Confidentiality of Alcohol and Other Drug Abuse Patient Records, 42 CFR Part 2, and cannot be disclosed without my written consent unless otherwise provided for in the regulations. I also understand that I may revoke this consent at any time except to the extent that action has been taken in reliance on it, and that in any event this consent expires automatically as follows:

_____
(Specification of the date, event, or condition upon which this consent expires)

Dated: _____   _____
Signature of patient

_____
Signature of parent, guardian, or authorized representative when required

---

Exceptions to Confidentiality Laws

Among the few exceptions to the laws are communications among staff members within a clinic, when they <u>must</u> share information to provide services to patients. Patient-identifying information may also be disclosed to medical personnel needing it to treat a medical emergency; however, the medical emergency exception may not be invoked to disclose such information to patients' families or other nonmedical personnel.[113]

Further details are given in DHHS Publication SMA-95-3018, *Confidentiality of Patient Records for Alcohol and Other Drug Treatment,* available from NCADI: 1-800-729-6686 or 1-301-468-2600.

Legal and ethical issues involved in treating adolescents who misuse alcohol are discussed in DHHS Publication SMA-93-2010, *Guidelines for the Treatment of Alcohol- and Other Drug-Abusing Adolescents,* also available from NCADI.

Chapter Summary

1. In this course, intervention refers to a planned clinical interaction with patients who misuse alcohol.

2. The goals of diagnostic assessments are: to obtain a diagnosis, determine the severity of patients' alcohol misuse, and determine patients' potential for rehabilitation.

3. When assessment interviews do not lead to <u>certain</u> diagnoses, clinicians should consider gathering more diagnostic data by convening a family meeting at the clinic (the patient must agree to and be present at the meeting).

4. Before patients can accept diagnoses of alcohol abuse or dependence, they must first overcome their denial of alcohol misuse, realize the consequences of their drinking habits, and decide to accept help.

5. When using benevolent coercion, clinicians must demonstrate genuine concern for patients and:
    a. Carefully explain clinical findings.
    b. Make sure patients understand both the findings and the fact that they indicate alcohol misuse.
    c. Explain to patients that current disorders will only worsen with continued alcohol misuse.

6. The option of moderate drinking can be used to motivate patients diagnosed with alcohol abuse (<u>not</u> alcohol dependence).

7. Addiction treatment settings include inpatient with intensive, highly structured care, and outpatient with either intensive or regular care.

8. All offices and clinics should have lists of current referral telephone numbers for sources of alcohol misuse treatment.

9. If clinicians decide to make any referral calls themselves, even with patients present, they <u>must</u> first obtain patients' written consent on a form meeting federal regulations.

Chapter 8   Alcohol and the Nervous System

Alcohol consumption can result in pleasurable effects (e.g., lowered inhibitions and relaxation) and disagreeable, even dangerous, effects (e.g., panic attacks and cognitive impairments). These effects occur, in part, because alcohol can directly or indirectly modify the synthesis and functions of neurotransmitters, highly specific chemicals which relay messages from one neuron (or nerve cell) to another. However, researchers studying neurotransmitter theory are finding that the effects of alcohol are far more complex than previously thought, and require further investigation.

Components of the Nervous System

The nervous system operates in an intricate, interactive fashion:

1. The central nervous system (CNS) component, comprising the brain and spinal cord, integrates body functions at both the conscious and subconscious levels; the CNS interprets and reacts to information it receives from the peripheral nervous system (PNS)

2. The PNS component, comprising all nerve fibers lying outside the brain and spinal cord, conducts information to and from the CNS; some of these fibers sense pain and temperature; others control muscular and excretory functions.[114]

Fig. 9 shows the basic unit of the nervous system, the neuron.[115] For the nervous system to do its job, myriad neurons must send signals to one another. Unfortunately, alcohol interferes with communication between neurons.[116]

Communication Between Neurons

A neuron's dendrites (*Fig. 9, top*) generally receive incoming messages, which they conduct toward the cell body. A change in electrical potential occurs, and, when it is positive, the neuron "fires," transmitting impulses along its axon at speeds up to several hundred miles an hour. Upon reaching the axon's branched terminals, the impulses cause vesicles to release neurotransmitters (chemical messengers) into the synapse, a microscopic gap between neurons. The neurotransmitters cross the synapse to bind to protein molecules called receptors on an adjacent neuron (electrical impulses cannot cross the synapse). Each receptor is shaped so that it binds with only one specific neurotransmitter, like a key fits into a lock.[2]

The chemical makeup of the neurotransmitter binding with a receptor determines the resultant effect, which can be:

1. Excitatory; e.g., acetylcholine, opioid, and glutamic acid neurotransmitters trigger electrical impulses in an adjacent neuron
2. Inhibitory; e.g., serotonin and gamma-aminobutyric acid (GABA) neurotransmitters reduce an adjacent neuron's sensitivity to other incoming messages
3. Excitatory or inhibitory; e.g., norepinephrine.[2,116]

This very limited information about the nervous system paves the way for subsequent discussions of mental disorders in which alcohol misuse affects neurotransmitter functioning, and medications which target either neurotransmitters or receptors.

Chapter Summary

1. The central nervous system (CNS), comprising the brain and spinal cord, interprets and reacts to information it receives from the peripheral nervous system.

2. The PNS, comprising all nerve fibers lying outside the brain and spinal cord, conducts information to and from the CNS.

3. The basic unit of the nervous system is the neuron (or nerve cell), which sends messages to, and receives them from, other neurons.

4. Neurons release neurotransmitters, which either excite or inhibit adjacent neurons; in the human body, alcohol can modify the synthesis and functions of neurotransmitters.

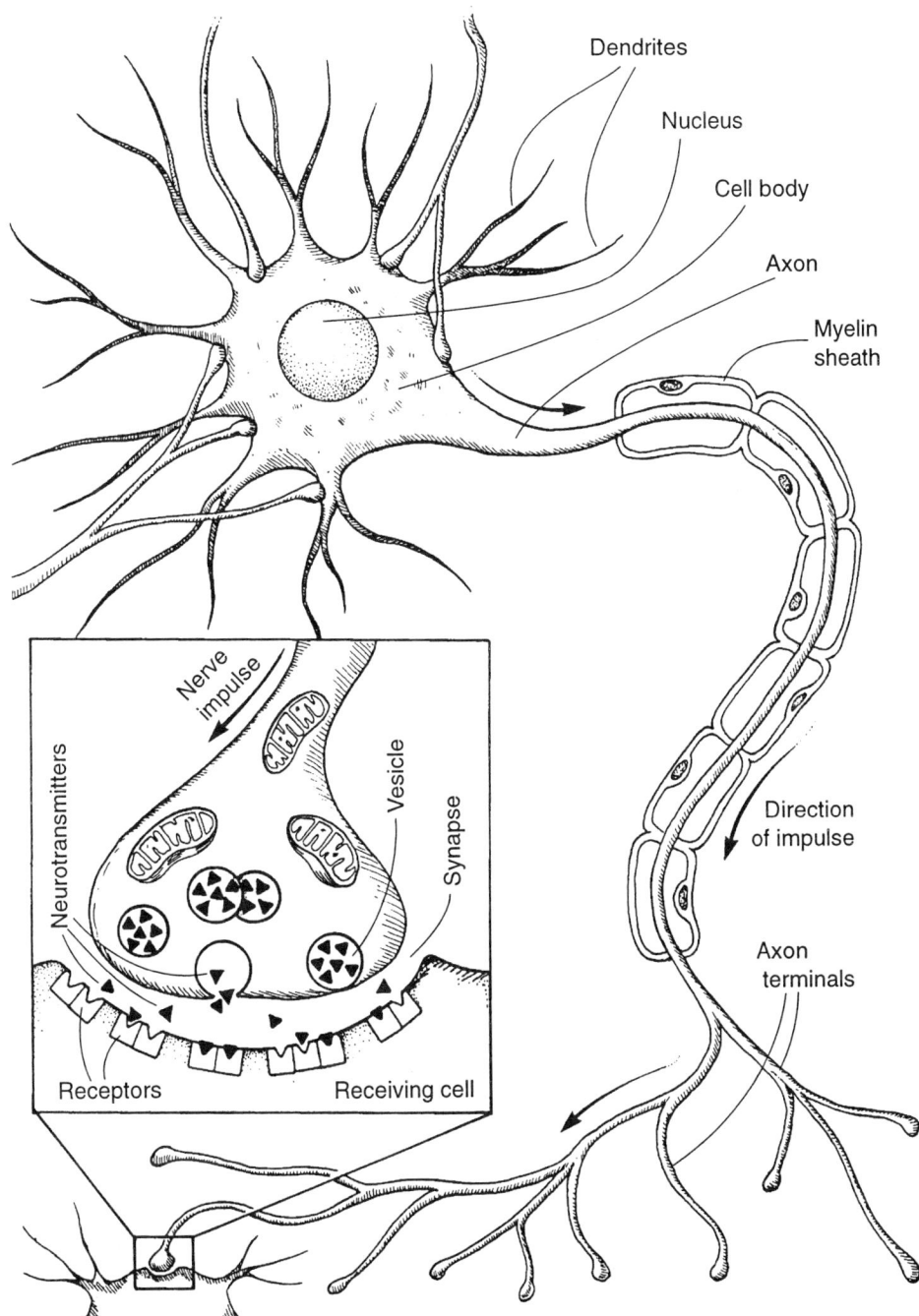

Fig. 9. How a Neuron Communicates. A branched dendrite (*top*) is often the neuronal part receiving a chemical message, delivered by a neurotransmitter from another neuron. An excitatory messenger (neurotransmitter) causes a receiving neuron to "fire" an electrical impulse along its tail-like axon and into terminals containing other neurotransmitters (*triangles in the inset*). These neurotransmitters are released into the synapse and move toward an adjacent neuron, where receptors on dendrites or other neuronal parts await their arrival.   *Drawing by Lydia Kubiuk*

Progress Test D (Chapters 7 & 8)

1. Even brief _____ _____ can reduce patient drinking.

2. The goals of diagnostic _____ are to obtain a diagnosis, assess the severity of alcohol misuse, and determine patients' potential for rehabilitation.

3. Patients may respond to _____ of alcohol abuse or dependence with agitation, anger, sulking, or silence.

4. Patients are _____ _____ for changing their behavior, and their readiness to make such changes varies greatly.

5. Types of addiction treatment settings include intensive-care inpatient, or _____-care or _____-care outpatient.

6. All offices and clinics should have lists of current _____ telephone numbers for sources of treatment of alcohol misuse and related disorders.

7. Confidentiality allows patients to determine _____ and ___ _____ information about their diagnoses and treatment may be disclosed.

8. Alcohol interferes with communication between _____.

9. _____ neurotransmitters trigger electrical impulses in an adjacent neuron; _____ neurotransmitters reduce an adjacent neuron's sensitivity to other incoming messages.

Chapter 9   Psychologic and Neurologic Disorders

Patients who misuse alcohol often report a variety of psychologic symptoms, which clinicians must sort out to determine the true cause. This chapter discusses psychologic and neurologic disorders, which are:

1. <u>Secondary</u> to alcohol abuse or dependence, and characterized as:
   a. <u>Transient</u> — exist during intoxication and alcohol withdrawal syndrome (AWS)
   b. <u>Persistent</u> — develop progressively as a result of chronic alcohol misuse
2. <u>Primary</u> and neither alcohol-induced nor due to a physiologic condition.

Transient Disorders

Algorithm 3 summarizes DSM-IV criteria for alcohol-induced mental disorders which can affect drinkers while they are intoxicated or undergoing AWS. Diagnosis of these <u>transient</u> disorders is difficult because many symptoms also apply to certain <u>primary</u> mental disorders.[74]

> When their BACs increase, drinkers become intoxicated and experience psychologic effects.

When their BACs increase, drinkers become intoxicated and experience psychologic effects. (*See Table 10, Chapter 4.*) Such effects in drinkers with BACs of <0.25 g/dL usually involve mood changes and motor impairment, do not require clinical care, and disappear several hours after the persons stop drinking. Even the more severe disorders shown in Algorithm 3 require only monitoring of the intoxicated persons' safety until these disorders disappear. However, when BACs are ≥0.25 g/dL, physiologic disorders (unconsciousness and reduced vital signs) outweigh intoxication's psychologic effects; these <u>demand</u> clinical care. (*See Transient Disorders, Chapter 10.*)

When people cease drinking, their bodies metabolize any remaining alcohol and, as their BACs decrease, they undergo alcohol withdrawal. Persons who occasionally consume excessive amounts of alcohol may suffer a mild form of withdrawal called the "hangover." (*See Transient Disorders, Chapter 10.*) On the other hand, chronic drinkers who cease or drastically reduce their alcohol consumption undergo AWS, an acute process which <u>must be</u> clinically monitored. These patients can also have one or more of the alcohol-induced mental disorders described in Algorithm 3. Generally, these disorders disappear when patients are detoxified and abstain from alcohol; however, some chronic drinkers have <u>protracted</u> withdrawals.[117] (*See Sedation Monitoring, Chapter 12.*)

Algorithm 3. Transient Mental Disorders		
(For complete diagnostic criteria, consult DSM-IV)		
If patient exhibits or has 1 or more of following: • Excessive anxiety • Panic attacks • Obsessions or compulsions • Clinically significant distress or impaired functioning	**And symptoms are <u>not</u> due to:** • Primary anxiety disorders; e.g., panic disorder with agoraphobia (*See Algorithm 7.*) • Anxiety disorders or delirium induced by other drugs, or a physiologic condition	**Then consider:** • Alcohol-induced anxiety disorder, with onset during intoxication or withdrawal
If patient exhibits or has 1 or more of following: • Fluctuating disturbance of consciousness • Clinically significant cognitive changes (e.g., disorientation)	**And symptoms are <u>not</u> due to:** • Delirium or dementia induced by other drugs, or a physiologic condition	**Then consider:** • Alcohol intoxication delirium, or • Alcohol withdrawal delirium (often called "delirium tremens")
If patient exhibits or has 1 or more of following: • Depressed, elevated, expansive, or irritable mood • Clinically significant distress or impaired functioning	**And symptoms are <u>not</u> due to:** • Primary mood disorders; e.g., major depressive episode (*See Algorithm 8.*) • Mood disorders or delirium induced by other drugs, or a physiologic condition	**Then consider:** • Alcohol-induced mood disorder, with onset during intoxication or withdrawal
If patient exhibits: • Delusions (or hallucinations <u>if</u> patients do not realize that they are alcohol-induced)	**And symptoms are <u>not</u> due to:** • Primary psychotic disorders; e.g., schizophrenia • Delirium induced by other drugs, or a physiologic condition • Head trauma, brain disorders, poisonings, or other neurologic conditions	**Then consider:** • Alcohol-induced psychotic disorder, with onset during intoxication or withdrawal

Adapted, and reprinted with permission, from the Diagnostic and Statistical Manual of Mental Disorders, *4th edition. Copyright 1994 American Psychiatric Association.*

Persistent Disorders

The more common, persistent mental and neurologic disorders secondary to chronic alcohol misuse are cirrhosis-related, nutrition-related, or of uncertain pathogenesis. Many of these grave disorders are characterized by brain lesions, neuronal death, and cognitive impairments.[118] Fig. 10 shows the various brain parts referred to in this chapter.

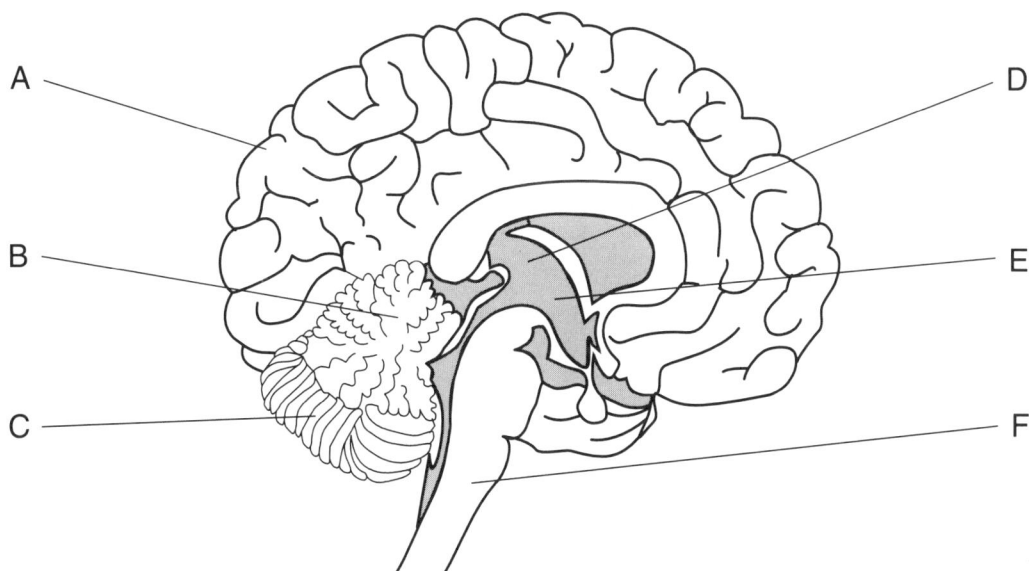

Fig. 10. Selected Brain Structures Damaged by Chronic Drinking

(A) The **cerebral cortex** controls and integrates sensory, motor, and higher mental functions (e.g., thinking, reason, emotion, and memory); it covers the cerebrum, the largest portion of the brain.

(B) The **vermis** separates the cerebellar hemispheres; upper lobules of the vermis are involved with refinement of coordination and postural stability of the legs and trunk; lower lobules support coordinated movement of the arms.

(C) The **cerebellum** (adj. cerebellar), the "little brain," is only about one-tenth the weight of the cerebrum, but contains about as many nerve cells (approximately 5 billion); it controls muscle tone, balance, and coordination.

(D) The **thalamus** relays sensory impulses to the cerebral cortex.

(E) The **hypothalamus** is involved with basic behavioral and physiologic functions.

(F) The **brain stem** connects the spinal cord to the cerebral hemispheres.

Portal-Systemic Encephalopathy

Portal-systemic encephalopathy (PSE) is caused indirectly by alcoholic cirrhosis, a disease involving liver structural damage and dysfunctioning. (*See Liver Disease, Chapter 10.*) In a healthy liver, enzymes break down or transform toxic substances into less harmful products, which can be either returned into the circulation or excreted in urine. One of these toxins is ammonia, which is produced primarily as a degradation product in the metabolism of dietary proteins and their building blocks, the amino acids. Ammonia-rich blood from the intestinal region is transported to the liver through the portal vein. In the liver, the ammonia is transformed into urea, a less toxic substance which can be excreted safely with the urine.[118]

> PSE is characterized by progressively worsening cognitive and neuro-muscular impairment.

Because a cirrhotic liver cannot detoxify normal amounts of ammonia, some of the toxin enters the general circulation and reaches the brain. Algorithm 4 shows that PSE is characterized by progressively worsening cognitive and neuromuscular impairment and, eventually, coma. This correlates with the belief that chronic brain exposure to excess ammonia interferes with functioning of certain neurotransmitters and their receptors, including glutamic acid (affecting learning and memory), serotonin (affecting mood and sleep), and dopamine (regulating movement and emotions). However, understanding of exactly how ammonia affects brain functions requires further study.[118]

Algorithm 4. Portal-Systemic Encephalopathy

If patient exhibits or has 1 or more of following:	Then clinician should test for:
• Stage 1. Abnormal sleep patterns, shortened attention span, irritability, apathy, tremor, incoordination • Stage 2. Personality changes, temporal disorientation, amnesia, asterixis, dysarthria, abnormal muscle tone • Stage 3. Confusion, drowsiness, paranoia, anger, stupor, hyperactive reflexes, muscle rigidity • Stage 4. Coma	• Alcoholic cirrhosis • Subtle signs of cognitive impairment **If PSE is confirmed, treatment could be:** • Counseling to motivate patient to abstain from alcohol • Ammonia-lowering drugs (lactulose or neomycin)—if cirrhosis is not severe • "Possible" liver transplant—if cirrhosis is severe

Because of its wide spectrum of signs and symptoms, PSE has been misdiagnosed as depression, schizophrenia, mild forms of mania, and Parkinson's disease. Diagnosis is further complicated by the fact that not all patients with PSE have obvious signs of liver disease or abnormal liver test results. Patients with less severe cirrhosis usually obtain PSE symptom relief by taking ammonia-lowering drugs.

Patients with severe cirrhosis should undergo serial neuropsychologic testing; with time, abnormal test results may indicate impairment of certain cognitive and motor performance skills (e.g., those involved in driving an automobile). These patients' PSE symptoms can be reversed, to some extent, by restoration of normal liver function (e.g., through a liver transplant);[118] however, in November 1996, the United Network for Organ Sharing (UNOS) ruled that patients with acute (not chronic) liver malfunction will be given top priority for transplants.

Wernicke-Korsakoff Syndrome

The neurologic disorder most commonly associated with chronic drinking is Wernicke-Korsakoff syndrome (WKS), a combination of Wernicke's encephalopathy and Korsakoff psychosis. Algorithm 5 shows WKS signs and symptoms, which patients may experience simultaneously.[75,119]

Algorithm 5. Wernicke-Korsakoff Syndrome	
If patient exhibits or has 1 or more of following:	**Then clinician should test/observe for:**
• Global confusional state (characterized by apathy, lethargy, drowsiness, disorientation, and impaired awareness or perceptual function) • Severe leg ataxia (characterized by feet wide apart, arms away from body, unstable trunk tilted forward, eyes fixed on ground, and rhythmic head tremor) • Nystagmus; sixth (abducens) nerve palsy • Amnesia (anterograde and/or retrograde); confabulation • Brain lesions in the thalamus, hypothalamus, cerebellum, vermis, and/or brain stem	• Wernicke encephalopathy • Korsakoff psychosis **If either of above are confirmed, treatment could be:** • Good nutrition and supplemental thiamine • Counseling to motivate patient to abstain from alcohol

WKS is caused by vitamin B_1 (thiamine) deficiency. Alcohol-dependent persons, after not eating for days, may eat only food high in carbohydrates and low in thiamine; enzymes breaking down carbohydrates use thiamine, thus depleting already low thiamine levels. In addition, alcohol damages the intestinal lining, which therefore absorbs little or no thiamine, depriving the brain of this critical nutrient. The amount of thiamine normally reaching the brain appears to exceed only slightly the amount required for proper brain functioning. Consequently, any reduction in thiamine availability can seriously affect brain metabolism and may cause brain lesions and cognitive dysfunction.[119]

> Any reduction in thiamine availability can seriously affect brain metabolism and may cause brain lesions and cognitive dysfunction.

If chronic alcohol misuse affects the functioning or structure of the cerebellum or vermis, patients can develop motor disorders such as ataxia and abnormal eye movement. Following treatment with thiamine, patients with acute-onset ataxia (as a component of Wernicke's encephalopathy) have about a 50% recovery rate; a smaller percentage of patients with subacute-onset ataxia (developed gradually as an isolated disorder) improve significantly.[117]

After thiamine treatment, however, approximately 50% to 65% of Wernicke's encephalopathy patients still have Korsakoff psychosis, a severe amnesia. Typically, onset of Korsakoff psychosis (called alcohol-induced persisting amnestic disorder in *DSM-IV)* is abrupt, affecting persons >40 years of age with histories of chronic alcohol use. These patients are severely impaired, occupationally and socially, and may require lifelong custodial care.[74]

Confabulation, the unconscious fabrication of stories by patients to fill in memory gaps, is the cardinal feature of Korsakoff psychosis. Another striking feature is anterograde amnesia; e.g., patients may need weeks of practice to learn the route from their hospital rooms to the cafeteria. Prolonged thiamine treatment, along with abstention from alcohol, has improved memory functions in some patients.[119] However, Victor's[75] studies showed a high mortality rate among patients with WKS: 20% died in the early stages of the disease and 17% in the chronic stages. Common causes of death were liver disorders, bacterial infections, and myocardial infarction.

Alcoholic Peripheral Neuropathy

Algorithm 6 shows selected signs and symptoms of alcoholic peripheral neuropathy (or alcoholic polyneuropathy). The disorder, also called neuropathic beriberi, is caused by thiamine deficiency.[75,117]

Algorithm 6. Alcoholic Peripheral Neuropathy	
If patient exhibits or has 1 or more of the following: • Dull, constant ache in feet or legs • Leg weakness, accompanied by tendon reflex loss, e.g., Achilles tendon reflex • Tenderness of calf muscles • Paresthesia (subjective complaint of cold feet) • Dysesthesia (sensation of "burning" on soles of feet) • Excessive sweating of feet and hands • Symmetrical loss of sensation in toes and fingers • Symmetrical motor function loss, beginning in distal muscle groups	**Then clinician should check for:** • Peripheral neuropathy **If confirmed, treatment could be:** • Counseling to motivate patient to abstain from alcohol • Balanced diet; large daily doses of thiamine (orally if possible; otherwise, I.V. or I.M.) • Medication for pain: usually aspirin or acetaminophen; occasionally 15 to 30 mg dose of codeine <u>if</u> patient stops drinking (*See Table 19 for alcohol-medication interactions.*) • Relief of aching (due to immobility) by frequent, gentle massage and passive movement of limbs • Measures to prevent denervated muscle contracture and fixed joints: position soles firmly against a footboard to prevent shortening of heel cords; use padded, molded splints on limbs of severely paralyzed patients and turn patients frequently; use physical therapy measures as patients' conditions permit.

Peripheral neuropathy first affects the feet and legs, then the arms; about 25% of patients complain mainly of pain and paresthesia. Patients with severe dysesthesia may find it intolerable to stand, walk, or bear the weight of a bed sheet on their feet (which can be avoided by use of a cradle support over the legs to elevate bedclothes).[75]

The major effect of alcoholic peripheral neuropathy is the degeneration of peripheral nerve axons. Recovery from the disease is slow; patients with severe cases may see no improvement for several weeks and may be unable to walk unaided for a year.[75] If motor loss begins in proximal, rather than distal, muscle groups, alcoholic myopathy may also be present; peripheral neuropathy and alcoholic myopathy can coexist.[117]

Optic Neuropathy

Optic neuropathy (or tobacco-alcohol amblyopia), another nutrition-related disorder, occasionally affects chronic drinkers. Typically, these patients report blurring of vision, which has developed gradually over several days or weeks; they may also experience dizziness. Optic neuropathy causes degeneration of the optic nerves; signs include visual acuity reduction and bilateral, centrocecal scotoma. Except in the most severe cases, improvement occurs with good nutrition and vitamin B supplements; however, if not treated, the condition progresses to irreversible optic atrophy.[75,117]

Alcoholic Dementia

Dementia affects at least 8% of alcohol-dependent persons. Like WKS, it causes amnesia, but it also produces a global decline in intellectual functions (e.g., judgment and abstract thinking). Pathogenesis of alcoholic dementia is uncertain, but findings include patchy neuronal degeneration and loss throughout the cerebral cortex.[117] Cutting[120] reports that, compared with Korsakoff psychosis, alcoholic dementia involves a longer drinking history and fewer ocular abnormalities.[2]

Alcoholic dementia develops gradually, but not stepwise like multi-infarct dementia. Geller[117] reports that, because alcoholic dementia develops insidiously against a background of chronic inebriation, the patient's family may attribute it to drunkenness, and it may not be recognized until the patient is detoxified. Even then, clinicians must differentiate between dementia caused by chronic drinking and that caused by hypothyroidism, syphilis, vitamin B_{12} deficiency, CNS mass lesions, or an infection.[121]

Primary Disorders

Some patients have dual (or comorbid) disorders, e.g., primary panic disorder and alcohol dependence. The difficult task of diagnosing dual disorders should be done only by persons with appropriate clinical training and experience in diagnosis. Some symptoms of the primary mental disorders discussed below are similar to those induced by alcohol misuse. (*See Algorithm 3.*)

Anxiety Disorders

Alcohol-dependent patients dually diagnosed with primary anxiety disorders could, if necessary, be given antidepressants and buspirone (Buspar®); the latter appears to exert its antianxiety effect by increasing serotonin concentrations in the brain. Because of their abuse potential, benzodiazepines are contraindicated.[122,123] Patients with anxiety disorders should abstain from caffeine, diet pills, and alcohol, and receive coping skills therapy. (*See Chapter 13.*)

> Buspirone appears to exert its antianxiety effect by increasing serotonin concentrations in the brain.

Primary anxiety disorders often diagnosed dually with alcohol dependence include social phobia, obsessive-compulsive disorder, and panic disorder with agoraphobia; Algorithm 7 shows, as an example, DSM-IV diagnostic criteria for the last named.[74] Alcohol-dependent persons with primary panic disorder, a chronic, often debilitating anxiety disorder, may drink to alleviate the symptoms; researchers are investigating the use of the antidepressant imipramine (Tofranil®) to treat such patients.[122]

Algorithm 7. Panic Disorder With Agoraphobia
(For complete diagnostic criteria, consult DSM-IV)

If patient exhibits or has 1 or more of following:	And panic attacks are <u>not</u> due to:	Then consider:
1. Recurrent, unexpected panic attacks, during which at least 4 of the following develop abruptly: • Chills, hot flushes, sweating, trembling, dizziness, paresthesia, and/or nausea • Sensation of choking or shortness of breath • Palpitations or chest pain • Derealization or depersonalization • Fear of losing control or dying 2. Following a panic attack, at least 1 month of concern about its implications or about having another attack 3. Agoraphobia	• The direct effects of alcohol use • A physiologic condition • Another mental disorder	• Panic disorder with agoraphobia

Adapted from, and printed with permission, from the Diagnostic and Statistical Manual of Mental Disorders, *4th edition. Copyright 1994 American Psychiatric Association.*

Depressive Disorders

A number of alcohol-dependent persons have primary manic-depressive disorder, chronic low-grade depression, or a major depressive episode. Algorithm 8 summarizes, as an example, DSM-IV diagnostic criteria for a major depressive episode. Current studies of medications for treating alcohol-dependent patients with primary depression focus on imipramine and desipramine (Norpramin®), which affect the neurotransmitter norepinephrine, and fluoxetine (Prozac®) and sertraline (Zoloft®), which affect serotonin receptors.[122] (*See Neuroregulating Medications, Chapter 12.*)

Algorithm 8. Major Depressive Episode *(For complete diagnostic criteria, consult DSM-IV)*		
If patient exhibits or has 1 or more of following: 1. Depressed mood and/or loss of interest or pleasure, plus 5 of the following symptoms nearly every day during a 2-week period: • Significant weight gain or loss (when not dieting) • Insomnia or hypersomnia • Psychomotor agitation • Fatigue • Feelings of worthlessness or guilt • Diminished ability to think or concentrate • Suicide plan or attempt 2. Clinically significant distress and/or impaired social and occupational functioning	**And symptoms are <u>not</u> due to:** • The direct effects of alcohol use • A physiologic condition • Bereavement • A mixed manic and major depressive episode (*Refer to DSM-IV for criteria.*)	**Then consider:** • Major depressive episode

Adapted from, and printed with permission, from the Diagnostic and Statistical Manual of Mental Disorders, *4th edition. Copyright 1994 American Psychiatric Association.*

Integrated Treatment

In the past, dually diagnosed patients often fell through the cracks in the health care system, which failed to treat one or the other of their disorders. However, in today's managed health care systems, treatment is increasingly integrated; i.e., psychiatric and alcohol-dependence treatments are provided simultaneously by clinicians trained in treatment approaches of both fields. Studies of integrated programs show success rates comparable with those for alcohol-dependence treatment in general, thereby providing hope that the presence of a primary mental disorder need not prevent effective addiction treatment.[124]

When prescribing medications for treatment of primary mental disorders, clinicians must consider:

1. Possible drug interactions (*See Chapter 11.*)
2. Potential for abuse (e.g., studies have indicated that alcohol-dependent persons are more likely than non-alcohol-dependent persons to abuse benzodiazepines)
3. Whether the symptoms are actually caused by protracted AWS (e.g., Schuckit et al.'s[125] studies showed that 90% of patients improved spontaneously within weeks, even when their AWS symptoms met diagnostic criteria for a primary anxiety disorder).

Chapter Summary

1. Transient, alcohol-induced mental disorders, affecting drinkers during intoxication and alcohol withdrawal syndrome, are secondary to alcohol abuse or dependence.

2. Diagnosis of secondary anxiety, delirium, mood, and psychotic disorders is difficult because many symptoms also apply to certain primary mental disorders.

3. Persistent psychologic and neurologic disorders secondary to chronic alcohol misuse are related to cirrhosis and malnutrition.

4. Portal-systemic encephalopathy is characterized by progressively worsening cognitive and neuromuscular impairment and, eventually, hepatic coma.

5. Wernicke-Korsakoff syndrome (WKS), the neurologic disorder most commonly associated with chronic drinking, is a combination of Wernicke's encephalopathy and Korsakoff psychosis.

6. Peripheral neuropathy, which results in degeneration of peripheral nerve axons, severely affects the feet and legs.

7. Like WKS, alcoholic dementia causes amnesia, but it also produces a global decline in intellectual functions.

8. Some patients have dual (or comorbid) disorders, which can be diagnosed only by persons with appropriate clinical training and experience.

9. Alcohol-dependent patients dually diagnosed with primary anxiety disorders could, if necessary, be given antidepressants and buspirone.

10. Researchers are studying the use of imipramine, desipramine, fluoxetine, and sertraline for treatment of primary depression in alcohol-dependent patients.

11. In today's managed health care systems, psychiatric and alcohol-dependence treatments are increasingly integrated.

12. When prescribing medications for treatment of primary mental disorders, clinicians must consider:
    a. Possible drug interactions
    b. Potential for abuse
    c. Whether the symptoms are actually caused by protracted AWS.

Progress Test E (Chapter 9)

1. When their BACs increase, drinkers become _____ and experience psychologic effects.

2. Many persistent, alcohol-induced, mental and neurologic disorders are characterized by brain lesions, _____ death, and cognitive impairments.

3. PSE, caused indirectly by alcoholic _____, is sometimes misdiagnosed as depression, schizophrenia, mild mania, and Parkinson's disease.

4. WKS is caused by a deficiency of _____ ____ _____.

5. The major effect of alcoholic peripheral neuropathy is the degeneration of peripheral _____ _____.

6. Clinicians must differentiate between _____ _____, caused by chronic drinking, and that caused by hypothyroidism, syphilis, vitamin B_{12} deficiency, CNS mass lesions, or an infection.

7. Benzodiazepines are contraindicated for patients with primary anxiety disorders because of their _____ _____.

8. When treating patients with primary mental disorders and secondary alcohol dependence, clinicians must consider whether the symptoms are actually caused by _____ _____.

Chapter 10 Physiologic Disorders

Alcohol is soluble in both water and lipids, so it permeates all body tissues;[70] therefore, chronic drinking can harm virtually every organ and system in the body. The primary site of alcohol damage is the liver, but the cardiovascular and endocrine systems can also be adversely affected, as well as the body's overall ability to resist disease (e.g., periodontal and other microbial diseases) and heal.

> Of utmost importance is the early identification of signs and symptoms.

This chapter summarizes data on alcohol-related physiologic disorders and the signs/symptoms which patients may report or exhibit during the taking of histories or physical examinations. Depending on their training, clinicians will either treat or refer such patients to specialists for treatment of the disorders. Of utmost importance is the early identification of signs and symptoms, so that therapy can be initiated and preventive steps taken before alcohol-induced tissue damage becomes irreversible.[70]

Transient Disorders

Persons suffering a hangover can have a variety of symptoms, including headache, nausea, vomiting, dizziness, thirst, and tremor; symptom severity probably relates to the amount of alcohol consumed. Hangover symptoms require no clinical treatment.[126]

> Severe intoxication, producing unconsciousness or depressed respiration, demands immediate medical attention.

However, severe intoxication, producing unconsciousness or depressed respiration, demands immediate medical attention. These signs are more common in patients with BACs of >0.25 g/dL. (*See Table 10, Chapter 4.*) In such cases, the priorities are:

1. Establishing an adequate airway (e.g., if needed, begin artificial respiration or perform tracheal intubation)
2. Maintaining blood circulation (if no heart beat or blood pressure is detectable, external cardiac massage is required; if there is evidence of atrial fibrillation, use a defibrillator).[127]

After patients' respiration and circulation are stabilized, treatment includes giving intravenous fluids, starting an electrocardiogram (EKG) or rhythm strip to monitor cardiac irregularities, drawing blood for chemical analysis, collecting urine for a toxicologic screen, and evaluating breath odor.[127] If alcohol overdose is suspected, a gastric lavage is done. If patients need medications, the potential for life-threatening interactions with alcohol <u>must</u> be assessed. (*See Chapter 11.*)

> If patients need medications, the potential for life-threatening interactions with alcohol must be assessed.

Severe alcohol intoxication produces nystagmus, which may persist for ≥6 hours.[128] Many intoxicated persons also suffer trauma, including spinal cord injuries and epidural hematomas, caused by falls and other accidents. (*For physiologic signs/symptoms of alcohol withdrawal syndrome, see Algorithm 11, Chapter 12.*)

Nutritional Problems

Alcohol provides calories (combustion of ethanol in a calorimeter yields 7 kcal/g);[129] however, Colditz et al.[130] report that, despite their high caloric intake, drinkers are no more obese than nondrinkers. In other studies, when alcohol was substituted for carbohydrates, subjects actually tended to lose weight, indicating they derived less energy from alcohol than from carbohydrates.[131] One reason for this inefficient alcohol-to-energy conversion may be the fact that much of the energy produced by the MEOS, triggered by chronic drinking, is lost as heat.[132] (*See Metabolism, Chapter 4.*)

> Despite high caloric intake, drinkers are no more obese than nondrinkers.

Drinkers who obtain approximately 25% or more of their total daily calories from alcohol are likely to have a deficient nutrient intake because they are neglecting important foods. Alcoholic beverages have extremely low protein and vitamin content (e.g., to satisfy daily protein needs, a person would have to drink 15 to 20 liters of beer; for thiamine needs, 25 liters). The carbohydrate content varies greatly, ranging from zero for vodka and whisky to about 120 g/L for sweetened wines.[129]

Furthermore, the body's use of the food chronic drinkers do eat is altered by alcohol, which:

1. Decreases secretion of digestive enzymes from the pancreas, thereby inhibiting the breakdown of nutrients into usable molecules
2. Damages cells lining the stomach and intestines, thereby impairing nutrient absorption (*See also Wernicke-Korsakoff Syndrome, Chapter 9.*)

3. Alters the transport, storage, and excretion of digested and absorbed nutrients, thereby preventing their full utilization (e.g., decreasing liver stores of vitamin A and increasing excretion of fat)
4. Impairs mechanisms by which the body controls blood glucose levels, resulting in either hyperglycemia or hypoglycemia.[132]

Patient Assessment and Treatment

From patients consuming >2 alcoholic drinks per day, dietary information can be obtained by:

1. Taking a dietary history and evaluating the amounts and types of foods being eaten
2. Taking body measurements such as weight, height, and skin-fold thickness to estimate fat reserves
3. Analyzing blood to measure circulating proteins, vitamins, and minerals.[132]

The best treatment for malnourished alcohol-dependent patients is adequate diet and abstention from alcohol. When nutritional supplements are used, dosages must not exceed normally prescribed levels if there is a possibility of overdose (e.g., vitamin A).[132] Table 17 shows nutritional therapy for alcohol-dependent patients, as recommended by Feinman and Lieber.[129]

Table 17. Nutritional Therapy for Alcohol-Dependent Patients	
Nutrient	**Comments**
Vitamin B$_1$ (thiamine)	Give 50 mg/day orally, I.M., or I.V.
Vitamin B$_2$ (riboflavin) and Vitamin B$_6$ (pyridoxine)	Give standard multivitamin preparations orally
Vitamin B$_9$ (folic acid)	Replace via hospital diet; if deficiency is severe, give orally or I.M.
Vitamin A	Give orally or I.M., only if deficiency is clearly diagnosed and abstinence from alcohol is assured
Zinc	Give I.V. for night blindness not responding to vitamin A replacement
Magnesium	Give to symptomatic patients with low blood serum magnesium
Iron	Give orally, I.M., or I.V., only if deficiency is clearly diagnosed
Calories and protein	Provide 25 to 35 kcal, and 1 to 1.25 g protein/kg ideal body weight

Digestive and Cardiovascular Disorders

Algorithm 9 gives a sampling of digestive and cardiovascular system disorders which can result from alcohol misuse.[90] Clinicians identifying these signs and/or symptoms should refer patients to specialists who, in turn, should work with those treating patients' alcohol abuse or dependence. All such patients must immediately abstain from alcohol; basic treatment involves care for AWS and malnutrition.

Gastrointestinal Disease

Algorithm 9 describes esophageal and stomach disorders related to misuse of alcohol, an irritant of mucosa. Incidence of esophagitis is high, and acute consumption of alcohol can cause gastroesophageal reflux. Early endoscopic visualization of the upper gastrointestinal (GI) tract should be performed on bleeding chronic drinkers.[133] Beta-blockers can be given to patients with known esophageal varices to prevent hemorrhaging.[121]

> Early endoscopic visualization of the upper GI tract should be performed on bleeding chronic drinkers.

Korsten and Lieber[133] report that antacids and histamine H_2-receptor antagonists do not alter the course of alcoholic gastritis, and that bleeding caused by gastric erosion tends to subside spontaneously. A recent report documents development of severe hepatocellular disease in alcohol-dependent patients with gastritis who used acetaminophen excessively.[89] Alcohol does not cause peptic ulcers; however, alcohol may exacerbate existing ulcers in smokers.[121]

Liver Disease

Because it is the primary site for alcohol metabolism, the liver is particularly vulnerable to alcohol's toxic effects, even in the absence of dietary deficiencies. Alcohol-induced liver disease often takes the following course: (1) fatty liver, followed by (2) early fibrosis and, possibly, alcoholic hepatitis, (3) severe fibrosis, and (4) cirrhosis.[70]

Fatty liver (or steatosis), a reversible disorder, is an accumulation of triglycerides and other fats in liver cells; it may be asymptomatic or associated with nonspecific symptoms. (*See Algorithm 9.*) Although fatty liver can be caused by obesity, diabetes mellitus, and several other disorders, most cases in the United States and Europe are the result of chronic drinking.

Alcoholic hepatitis, which affects patients with varying severity, is diagnosed by needle liver biopsy. Liver cells are swollen with granular cytoplasm, due to an increase in cytosolic proteins. Signs

AWS- Alcohol Withdrawal Syndrome

distinguishing acute alcoholic hepatitis from acute viral hepatitis are florid vascular spiders, a greatly enlarged liver, and leukocytosis. In 50% of patients, an arterial murmur may be heard over the liver. Histologic cholestasis indicates a bad prognosis for this disorder. Sherlock and Dooley[134] report that 20% to 50% of patients with acute alcoholic hepatitis die.

Fibrosis, replacement of healthy liver tissue with scar tissue, is caused by necrosis and inflammation; it may also occur because alcohol affects liver lipocytes (or fat-storing cells). Chronic alcohol consumption transforms lipocytes into cells which produce collagen, the characteristic protein of fibrous tissues. In the pre-cirrhosis stage of liver disease, agents which replenish reduced glutathione can be effective.[70]

Algorithm 9. Digestive and Cardiovascular System Disorders

If patient exhibits or has 1 or more of following:	Then clinician should test for:	If confirmed, some therapeutic considerations are:
Dysphagia, chest pain ("heartburn"), vomiting of blood, weight loss	Esophageal disorders: • Chronic esophagitis • Malignancies • Mallory-Weiss tears • Varices	• Provide sclerotherapy for esophageal variceal hemorrhage[121]
Gas, bloating, heartburn, nausea	Gastritis: • Chronic • Acute hemorrhagic	• Give antibiotics if infection with *Helicobacter pylori* is present in chronic gastritis[121] • Stabilize patient and correct clotting abnormalities (e.g., with vitamin K, fresh frozen plasma, and platelets) for acute hemorrhagic gastritis[133]
Mild abdominal discomfort, anorexia	Fatty liver (or alcoholic steatosis)	• Consider giving anabolic steroids, but their benefits must be balanced against their cholestatic potential[133]
Fever, nausea, vomiting, abdominal pain, enlarged liver, jaundice, florid vascular spiders, leukocytosis	Acute alcoholic hepatitis	• Consider giving prednisolone if encephalopathy is present; it has decreased short-term mortality in clinical trials[134]
Weight loss, bleeding abnormalities, edema, enlarged liver	Alcoholic cirrhosis	• Consider "possible" liver transplant, for patients who remain abstinent for 6 months[134]
Intense abdominal pain, nausea, vomiting, fever	Acute pancreatitis	• Give I.V. fluids (nothing orally; patients need bowel rest)
Intractable abdominal pain, weight loss, diarrhea	Chronic pancreatitis	• Give oral hypoglycemic drugs (mild cases) or insulin if patient has stopped drinking (*See Table 19, Chapter 11, for drug interactions.*) • Pancreatic enzyme replacement
Fatigue, hypertension, palpitations, shortness of breath, cardiac arrhythmias, chronic cardiomyopathy, ischemic or hemorrhagic stroke	Cardiovascular and cerebrovascular disorders	• Give anticoagulants, diuretics, venodilators, and arteriolar vasodilators for cardiomyopathy; however, these patients may have increased sensitivity to digitalis[133]

Alcoholic cirrhosis, which is irreversible, is caused by an imbalance between the production and the degradation of collagen.[70] Cirrhosis is characterized by fibrosis, nodules, and loss of normal structure of liver tissue, accompanied by functional decline.[2] Therapy is directed at the complications of cirrhosis: portal hypertension, encephalopathy, and ascites.[134] Alcohol-related cirrhosis has been associated with development of primary liver cancer (or hepatoma).[90]

> Persons with cirrhosis may have life expectancies an estimated 9 to 22 years lower than the average.

Among chronic, alcohol-related physiologic disorders, cirrhosis is the leading cause of death.[5] It is responsible not only for increased mortality, but for premature mortality: persons with this disease may have life expectancies an estimated 9 to 22 years lower than the average.[2]

Alcoholic Pancreatitis

Researchers are not sure how alcohol affects functioning of the pancreas, but they have proposed theories on how pancreatic injury occurs. Acute pancreatitis is characterized by destruction of the membranes of pancreatic acinar cells; such cell injury may lead to interstitial leaking of digestive enzymes secreted by the cells. Singh[135] reports that proteolytic activities of these enzymes may cause "autodigestion" of tissue. Chronic pancreatitis is more commonly associated with alcohol dependence than is acute pancreatitis. Korsten[136] reports that relapsing pancreatitis in chronic drinkers may be due to an increase in protein content of pancreatic secretions, which induces the formation of viscous protein plugs in pancreatic ducts.

Algorithm 9 shows therapeutic considerations for alcoholic pancreatitis. Pancreatic enzyme replacements may resolve vitamin deficiency, stimulate weight gain, and reduce chronic pain.[121]

Cardiovascular Disease

Alcohol's vasopressor effect is linked to hypertension in chronic drinkers. Control of hypertension requires abstinence from alcohol and, if abstinence does not reverse the hypertension, compliance with antihypertensive therapy.[133]

Chronic alcohol misuse can cause cardiomyopathy, characterized by a dilated, weakened heart muscle. In the end stages of the disease, which affects both chambers of the heart, dysfunction of the left ventricular chamber of the heart may lead to pulmonary hypertension (increase in blood pressure in the lung vessels) and can then cause right-sided heart failure. Because alcohol-induced cardiomyopathy is clinically and pathologically indistinguishable from other forms of congestive cardiomyopathy, its diagnosis depends on knowledge of a patient's history of alcohol misuse.[2]

Binge drinking, as well as chronic alcohol consumption, can cause arrhythmias, explaining in part the high incidence of sudden death of alcohol-dependent persons. Atrial fibrillation and ventricular dysrhythmia are also commonly associated with alcohol misuse.[2]

> Very heavy drinking has been associated with a fourfold increase in the risk of hemorrhagic stroke.

<u>Very</u> heavy drinking (about 5 drinks per day) has been associated with a fourfold increase in the risk of hemorrhagic stroke, as well as increased risk of ischemic stroke. Moderate drinking (1 or 2 drinks per day) could possibly decrease risk of ischemic stroke.[2] For some persons, moderate alcohol consumption raises the level of high-density lipoproteins; however, the same apparent protective effect against coronary artery disease has been found in people who consume only 1 drink per week or per month.[70] Any benefits may still be outweighed by other alcohol-related complications: risk of strokes caused by bleeding, impaired driving skills caused by fatigue or drugs which increase alcohol's effect, and alcohol's interference with functions of medications used to treat severe heart disease.[63]

Oral Disorders

Enlarged parotid glands and alterations in salivary secretion are common in patients with alcoholic cirrhosis. Glossitis and stomatitis in alcohol-dependent patients usually respond to supplementary vitamin B complex and folate. Such patients, particularly if they smoke, also have increased incidence of oropharyngeal cancer; because this malignancy usually does not metastasize to distant sites, early detection and curative resection are vital.[133,137] Alcohol-dependent persons may also exhibit oral signs and symptoms listed in Table 14. (*See Chapter 6.*)

> Compromise of liver function by alcohol can result in altered metabolism of amide-class local anesthetics.

When planning invasive oral procedures for alcohol-dependent patients, dentists should first arrange for, then learn the results of, blood tests evaluating residual liver function. Compromise of liver function by alcohol can result in altered metabolism of amide-class local anesthetics (*see Table 19, Chapter 11*), and certain antibiotics, analgesics, and sedatives-hypnotics. Because less metabolism occurs in the liver with ester-class local anesthetics than with amides, the ADA recommends, <u>for</u> <u>patients</u> <u>with</u> <u>alcoholic</u> <u>cirrhosis</u>, use of 0.4% propoxycaine (Ravocaine®) combined with 2% procaine (Novocain®), available in 1.8 mL dental cartridges.[89] For most patients, however, the dental profession generally uses amides (e.g., lidocaine and mepivacaine) because of the significant number of allergic responses to ester-class local anesthetics.

Patients with alcoholic cirrhosis may also have deficient protein levels, which can impair clotting and increase the risk of intraoperative or postoperative hemorrhaging. In addition, alcohol suppresses bone marrow production of platelets (thrombocytopenia), which prolongs bleeding time. Alcohol also suppresses bone-marrow leukocyte production and/or causes produced leukocytes to function less efficiently. Therefore, chronic drinkers may heal more slowly after oral surgery, and be more susceptible to osteomyelitis.[89]

Gout Attacks

Alcohol misuse can trigger attacks of gout. This typically acute monarthritis affects the ankle, knee, or first metatarsophalangeal joint; however, other joints may be involved when the attacks are recurrent or when hyperuricemia, if present, is untreated. Intracellular crystals, which are needle-shaped and have strong negative birefringence (double refraction), characterize gout. Nonsteroidal anti-inflammatory drugs (e.g., indomethacin/Indocid®) are used to treat acute attacks of gout; colchicine, because of its side effects, and medications which alter uric acid levels in blood serum are contraindicated.[138]

Reproductive and Sexual Dysfunction
Endocrine Abnormalities

In men, alcohol directly reduces testosterone level; if prolonged, this condition may contribute to feminization of males' sexual characteristics; e.g., breast enlargement (or gynecomastia). Chronic alcohol misuse can also cause bilateral testicular atrophy, leading to some degree of infertility. Acute alcohol consumption is believed to affect release of hormones from the hypothalamus and pituitary; chronic, heavy alcohol consumption may also inhibit vitamin A metabolism, interfering with normal sperm structure and movement.[139,140]

In premenopausal women, chronic alcohol misuse can increase the risk of spontaneous abortions, and can disturb menstrual cycles (cycles are irregular or without ovulation, menstruation ceases, or menopause occurs early). Alcohol causes these dysfunctions either directly, by altering the amounts of reproductive hormones (e.g., progesterone and estrogens), or indirectly, as a result of malnutrition or liver or pancreatic disease.[139,141]

Postmenopausal women with a history of chronic alcohol misuse increase their risks for osteoporosis, because alcohol inhibits the activity of bone-forming cells and, by disturbing vitamin D metabolism, inhibits absorption of dietary calcium. However, studies suggest that consumption of small amounts of alcohol (3 to 6 drinks per week) may benefit postmenopausal women: alcohol can increase the conversion of testosterone into estradiol, an estrogen which, after menopause, normally declines drastically because it is no longer synthesized in the ovaries. Estradiol deficiency has been linked with increased risk for cardiovascular disease and osteoporosis. Research continues on which female subgroups truly benefit from some alcohol intake, and on what drinking levels are effective without increasing other risks.[139]

Fetal Alcohol Syndrome

Alcohol crosses the placenta and interferes with fetal development; this can lead to fetal alcohol syndrome (FAS) and other alcohol-related birth defects (ARBDs), which do not meet all FAS criteria. Table 18 shows possible anomalies of FAS; use of certain medications can also produce some of these problems. Low birth weight, averaging 37% below normal, is the anomaly most often reported in babies with FAS; however, whether they drink or not, women who smoke during pregnancy also tend to have small babies.[2,63,141,142]

Table 18. Possible Anomalies of Fetal Alcohol Syndrome	

• Low birth weight
• Slow growth after birth
• Mental retardation
• Heart murmur
• Birthmark
• Hernia
• Urinary tract abnormality
	• Head abnormalities:
	  • Small head circumference
	  • Indistinct philtrum (or groove in middle of upper lip)
	  • Low nasal bridge and short nose
	  • Thin upper lip
	  • Small eye openings (or short palpebral fissures) and skin folds at eye corners
	  • Elongated, flattened cheeks

Given the variety of anomalies associated with FAS and other ARBDs, it is impossible to determine a reliable threshold for safe alcohol consumption during pregnancy. Jacobson et al. found measurable increases in abnormal neurobehavioral tests for 1-year-olds whose mothers had consumed >1 alcoholic drink (>0.5 oz pure alcohol) per day while pregnant. Other studies have suggested that, for delayed mental development, attention deficits, or lower IQ scores, the threshold level is more than 7 drinks per week. Because it is impossible to determine which fetuses may be at risk for damage from low levels of alcohol exposure, the Surgeon General has recommended that all women abstain from drinking throughout pregnancy.[141,142]

Clinicians should advise pregnant patients who drink that, if they stop drinking, some alcohol-induced fetal development deficiencies can be avoided or ameliorated.[141] However, pregnant patients with tolerance to alcohol should undergo AWS <u>under medical supervision</u>, including collaboration with an obstetrician. Sudden cessation of drinking can cause life-threatening disorders in both the mother and the fetus, and medications may be needed to control the withdrawal.[143] (*See Table 20, Chapter 12.*)

Chapter Summary

1. Chronic drinking can harm virtually every body organ and system, because alcohol permeates all body tissues.

2. Severe intoxication, producing unconsciousness or depressed respiration, requires immediate medical attention.

3. Alcohol provides calories, but alcohol-to-energy conversion is inefficient, perhaps because much of it is lost as heat.

4. Patients with digestive and/or cardiovascular system disorders must immediately abstain from alcohol, then be treated for AWS and malnutrition.

5. Alcohol does not cause peptic ulcers; however, alcohol may exacerbate existing ulcers in smokers.

6. Alcohol-induced liver disease often begins with (1) fatty liver, followed by (2) early fibrosis and, possibly alcoholic hepatitis, (3) severe fibrosis, and (4) cirrhosis.

7. Signs distinguishing acute alcoholic hepatitis from viral hepatitis are florid vascular spiders, an enlarged liver, and leukocytosis.

8. Alcoholic cirrhosis, which is irreversible, is caused by an imbalance between the production and degradation of collagen.

9. Chronic pancreatitis is more commonly associated with alcohol dependence than is acute pancreatitis.

10. Because alcohol-induced cardiomyopathy is indistinguishable from other forms of congestive cardiomyopathy, its diagnosis depends on knowledge of a patient's history of alcohol misuse.

11. When planning invasive oral procedures for alcohol-dependent patients, dentists should first arrange for, then learn the results of, blood tests evaluating residual liver function.

12. The Surgeon General has recommended that <u>all</u> women abstain from drinking throughout pregnancy.

Chapter 11   Drug Interactions

When taking patient histories, clinicians should identify all drugs that patients are taking.

Alcohol is considered a drug (CNS depressant); its interactions with prescribed, over-the-counter, or illegal drugs are potentially dangerous. When taking patient histories, clinicians should identify all drugs that patients are taking and then advise them about potential interactions with alcohol. Astute clinicians, when suspecting that patients may be intoxicated, will avoid giving medications (even if it means postponing treatment) and explain that drug combinations might cause a medical emergency.

Alcohol and Medications

The interactions of many medications with alcohol can produce illness, injury, or death. Alcohol-medication interactions are a factor in an estimated 25% of all emergency room admissions. An unknown number of less alarming interactions may go unrecognized or unrecorded.[144]

More than 2,800 prescription medications are available in the United States, and physicians write 14 billion prescriptions annually; in addition, approximately 2,000 medications are available over the counter. Approximately 70% of the adult population consumes alcohol at least occasionally, and 10% consumes it daily. These combined statistics suggest that some concurrent use of alcohol and medications is inevitable.[144]

The elderly are especially likely to mix medications and alcohol.

About 10% of persons aged ≥60 in the United States meet the diagnostic criteria for alcohol abuse. Although persons aged ≥65 constitute only 12% of the U.S. population, they take 25% to 30% of all prescription medications. Therefore, the elderly are especially likely to mix medications and alcohol, and are at particular risk for the adverse consequences of such combinations. Compared with younger persons, the elderly are more likely to suffer drug side effects, which tend to intensify with advancing age.[144,145]

Guram et al.[146] report two types of alcohol-medication interactions, which overlap:

1. Because alcohol is a CNS depressant, synergistic (or additive) reactions occur when it is combined with sedatives/hypnotics (*See, e.g., diazepam and secobarbital in Table 19.*)

2. When alcohol is combined with medications metabolized in the liver, the medications' effects may be:
   a. Increased—setting patients up for exaggerated or overdose-like responses (*See, e.g., brompheniramine, codeine, and nitroglycerin in Table 19.*)
   b. Reduced—lessening therapeutic effects (*See, e.g., isoniazid and rifampin in Table 19.*)

> Alcohol's adverse interactions with antihistamines and benzodiazepines are well recognized.

Table 19 shows classes of medications, a partial list of generic and brand names, and changes alcohol causes in their effects/actions, which can vary greatly from one person to another. Although many types of medications interact adversely with alcohol, the reactions with antihistamines and benzodiazepines are well recognized.[146]

Alcohol and Illegal Drugs

Alcohol and cocaine are often used together because alcohol lessens the anxiety and sleep disruption caused by cocaine. Concurrent use of alcohol and cocaine produces endogenous cocaethylene (or ethylcocaine), which enhances and extends the cocaine euphoria.[147] During clinical trials, administration of disulfiram (Antabuse®) to persons dependent on alcohol and cocaine substantially decreased their use of both drugs. Alcohol and opioids (e.g., heroin) are also often used together; the combination appears to be synergistic.[2] Many deaths are caused by concurrent use of alcohol and cocaine or opioids. (*See Emergencies and Deaths, Chapter 2.*)

Table 19. Alcohol-Medication Interactions

When prescribing or using:	Such as: (generic and brand name examples)	Be aware that:
Anesthetics (general)	Enflurane (Ethrane®) Halothane (Fluothane®) Propofol (Diprivan®)	• <u>Chronic</u> alcohol use increases (1) the risk of liver damage caused by enflurane and halothane, and (2) the propofol dose required to induce unconsciousness.
Anesthetics (local amide-class)	Lidocaine (L-Caine®, Lidoject®) Mepivacaine (Carbocaine®) Prilocaine (Citanest®)	• <u>Chronic</u> alcohol use, which compromises liver function, impairs amide metabolism; this can cause restlessness and tremor, which may proceed to convulsions.
Antibiotics	Furazolidone (Furoxone®) Griseofulvin (Grisactin®) Isoniazid (Isotamine®) Metronidazole (Flagyl®) Quinacrine (Atabrine®) Rifampin (Rifadin®)	• <u>Acute</u> alcohol use, combined with certain antibiotics, can cause nausea, vomiting, headache, and, on occasion, seizures. • <u>Acute</u> alcohol use reduces the effects of isoniazid. • <u>Chronic</u> alcohol use reduces the effects of rifampin.
Anticoagulants	Acenocoumarol (Sintrom®) Warfarin sodium (Coumadin®)	• <u>Acute</u> alcohol use intensifies the effects of anticoagulants and the risk of life-threatening hemorrhages. • <u>Chronic</u> alcohol use reduces the effects of anticoagulants.
Antidepressants (tricyclics)	Amitriptyline (Elavil®) Desipramine (Pertofrane®) Doxepin (Sinequan®) Imipramine (Tofranil®) Nortriptyline (Aventyl®)	• <u>Acute</u> alcohol use intensifies tricyclics' sedative effects. • <u>Chronic</u> alcohol use intensifies the effects of some tricyclics, even in recovering alcoholics.
Antidepressants (monoamine oxidase inhibitors—MAOIs)	Isocarboxazid (Marplan®) Phenelzine (Nardil®) Tranylcpromine (Parnate®)	• <u>Any</u> consumption (even one standard drink) of tyramine-containing beers and wines, combined with MAOI ingestion, may produce a hypertensive hyperpyrexic crisis.
Antidiabetics (oral hypoglycemics)	Acetohexamide (Dymelor®) Chlorpropamide (Diabinese®) Insulin (Iletin®) Tolazamide (Tolinase®) Tolbutamide (Orinase®)	• <u>Acute</u> alcohol use intensifies, and <u>chronic</u> alcohol use reduces, the effects of antidiabetics, which can cause either hypoglycemia or hyperglycemia. • <u>Any</u> alcohol use, combined with antidiabetics may produce nausea and headache.
Antihistamines	Brompheniramine (Dimetapp®) Chlorpheniramine (Coricidin®) Clemastine (Tavist®) Diphenhydramine (Benadryl®)	• <u>Any</u> alcohol use can intensify the sedative effect of antihistamines, and may cause excessive dizziness and sedation in older persons.
Antipsychotics	Chlorpromazine (Thorazine®) Prochlorperazine (Compazine®)	• <u>Acute</u> alcohol use intensifies the sedative effects of antipsychotics, resulting in incoordination and potentially fatal breathing difficulties. • <u>Chronic</u> alcohol use, combined with use of antipsychotics, may cause liver damage.

Table 19. Alcohol-Medication Interactions (Continued)

When prescribing or using:	Such as: (generic and brand name examples)	Be aware that:
Antiseizure medications	Carbamazepine (Tegretol®) Phenobarbital (Luminal®) Phenytoin (Dilantin®) Primidone (Mysoline®)	• <u>Any</u> alcohol use, combined with use of antiseizure medications, may enhance CNS depression. <u>Chronic</u> alcohol use can reduce the effects of antiseizure medications, even when drinkers have abstained for a lengthy period.
Cardiovascular medications	Guanethidine (Ismelin®) Hydralazine (Apresoline®) Methyldopa (Aldomet®) Nitroglycerin (Nitrosat®) Propranolol (Inderal®) Reserpine (Serpasil®)	• <u>Acute</u> alcohol use intensifies the blood-pressure lowering effects of cardiovascular medications, which can produce postural hypotension. • <u>Chronic</u> alcohol use reduces the blood-pressure lowering effects of propranolol.
Narcotic analgesics (opioids)	Codeine Meperidine (Demerol®) Morphine Opium (Pantopon®) Oxycodone (Percodan®) Pentazocine (Talwin®) Propoxyphene (Darvon®)	• <u>Any</u> alcohol use, combined with opioids, intensifies the sedative effects of both substances, increasing the risk of death.
Nonnarcotic analgesics OTC medications	Acetaminophen (Tylenol®) Aspirin (Alka-Seltzer®, Bayer Aspirin®, Bufferin®) Ibuprofen (Advil®)	• <u>Chronic</u> alcohol use transforms acetaminophen into chemicals which can cause liver damage; only 2.6 grams of acetaminophen can produce this effect. • <u>Any</u> alcohol use exacerbates aspirin-caused stomach bleeding; aspirin may intensify the effects of alcohol. • <u>Any</u> alcohol use with ibuprofen or aspirin exaggerates their tendency to prolong bleeding time.
Sedatives/hypnotics: benzodiazepines	Diazepam (Valium®) Flurazepam (Dalmane®) Lorazepam (Ativan®)	Any sedative-hypnotic can have a synergistic reaction with alcohol; therefore: • <u>Any</u> alcohol use, combined with benzodiazepines, may cause severe drowsiness (which can impair driving ability); it can also cause depressed heart and breathing functions.
Sedatives/hypnotics: barbiturates	Amobarbital (Amytal®) Pentobarbital (Nembutal®) Phenobarbital (Luminal®) Secobarbital (Seconal®)	Any sedative-hypnotic can have a synergistic reaction with alcohol; therefore: • <u>Any</u> alcohol use intensifies the sedative effects of barbiturates, sometimes leading to coma or fatal respiratory arrest.
Nonbarbiturate sedatives	Chloral hydrate (Chlorhydrate®) Meprobamate (Miltown®)	• <u>Any</u> alcohol use with these medications can be synergistic and result in CNS depression.

Chapter Summary

1. When taking patient histories, clinicians should identify all drugs (prescription, over-the-counter, and illegal) that patients are taking, then advise them about potential interactions with alcohol.

2. Alcohol-medication interactions are a factor in an estimated 25% of all emergency room admissions.

3. Compared with younger persons, the elderly are more likely to suffer drug side effects, which tend to intensify with advancing age.

4. Because alcohol is a CNS depressant, synergistic effects occur when it is combined with sedatives/hypnotics.

5. When alcohol is combined with medications metabolized in the liver, the medications' effects may be increased or reduced.

6. The adverse interactions of alcohol with antihistamines and benzodiazepines are well recognized.

7. Concurrent use of alcohol and cocaine produces endogenous cocaethylene, which enhances and extends the cocaine euphoria.

Progress Test F (Chapters 10 & 11)

1. Chronic drinking can damage almost every body organ and system because alcohol is soluble in both water and _____.

2. Severe intoxication is more likely to produce unconsciousness or depressed respiration in patients with BACs of _____.

3. Drinkers who get 25% or more of their total daily calories from alcohol are likely to have a deficient _____ _____.

4. Alcohol causes esophageal and stomach disorders because it irritates _____.

5. Alcoholic cirrhosis is an _____ liver disorder.

6. Hypertension in chronic drinkers is linked to alcohol's _____ effect.

7. The most common anomaly in babies with FAS is _____ _____ _____.

8. The _____ are especially likely to mix medications and alcohol, and are at particular risk for the adverse consequences of such combinations.

9. Any alcohol use exacerbates _____-caused stomach bleeding.

10. Sedatives-hypnotics can have a _____ reaction with alcohol.

Chapter 12 Pharmacotherapy

Alcohol-dependent patients entering treatment for addiction may require any of several types of pharmacotherapy to:

1. Alleviate severe alcohol withdrawal syndrome (AWS) signs and symptoms (e.g., by detoxification with sedatives-hypnotics)
2. Discourage drinking during rehabilitation (e.g., with aversive medications)
3. Reduce craving for alcohol (e.g., with neuroregulating medications).[112]

Withdrawal and Medical Detoxification

The majority of patients undergoing AWS will respond to reassurance and supportive measures, with no need of sedatives-hypnotics; those not responding to this approach can be sedated. The sedative-hypnotic of choice depends on the presence of various physiologic conditions. (*See Algorithm 10.*)[148]

Algorithm 10. Conditions Affecting Sedative-Hypnotic Choice	
If patient is:	**Clinicians could use:**
Suffering significant liver disease, which impairs metabolism of long-acting benzodiazepines	• The barbiturate phenobarbital (e.g., Luminal®), or • Shorter-acting benzodiazepines (e.g., oxazepam and lorazepam)
Prone to seizures unrelated to alcohol misuse	• A medication with anticonvulsive properties (phenobarbital, diazepam, or lorazepam)
Suffering alcoholic gastritis	• Lorazepam, diazepam, or phenobarbital I.M., or • Lorazepam sublingually
Pregnant	• See Table 20

Use of Sedatives-Hypnotics

Benzodiazepines such as diazepam (Valium®), chlordiazepoxide (Librium®), oxazepam (Serax®), and lorazepam (Ativan®) are widely used to treat AWS. These medications can cause temporary drowsiness, lethargy, and amnesia.[122,100] Clinicians <u>must</u> know patients' BACs before administering any sedatives-hypnotics, because using them to treat patients with high BACs can provoke a synergistic reaction with alcohol; this results in hypotension, shock, or coma. Benzer's[148] suggested rule of thumb is "to withhold medications for treating AWS symptoms while patients have BACs of >0.15 g/dL."

Algorithm 11 shows AWS signs and symptoms, stages, and treatments (using, e.g., chlordiazepoxide) for nonpregnant patients.[148] In mild cases of AWS, Stage I lasts only 24-48 hours; in severe cases, it lasts 3-5 days. Patients who are untreated, or inadequately treated, in Stage I, may suffer the more severe Stage II AWS, including hallucinations; a few patients reach the potentially life-threatening Stage III AWS, which includes delirium tremens.

Table 20 shows three possible sedation schedules, recommended by the Center for Substance Abuse Treatment (CSAT),[149] for pregnant patients undergoing alcohol withdrawal. Fetal well-being should be carefully monitored.[143]

Table 20. Sedation for Pregnant Patients With AWS		
Choices of Schedules	Doses/Duration	Comments
Phenobarbital	Initially, 15-60 mg orally every 4 to 6 hrs as needed for first 2 days; decreasing gradually to 15 mg by 4th day	• Can cause fetal or neonatal toxicity • Acts as a weak teratogen, sometimes causing minor craniofacial anomalies
Diazepam	10 mg every 2 hrs as needed, with max. of 150 mg/24 hrs; decreasing gradually at rate of 20% to 25% over 5 days	• Doses of ≥30 mg can cause fetal or neonatal toxicity • I.V. benzodiazepines can cause a rise in fetal or neonatal bilirubin levels, presenting a risk of kernicterus
Chlordiazepoxide	25-50 mg 4 times a day for first 2 days; decreasing gradually to 10 mg 4 times a day for days 8-10	Same as for diazepam

Recent research shows that AWS symptoms appear to result, at least in part, from overactivity of the neurons using the neurotransmitter norepinephrine; therefore, medications such as clonidine (Catapres®) and propranolol (Inderal®), which decrease norepinephrine activity, are also useful in treating AWS. Although these medications cause less mental confusion or sedation than benzodiazepines, they fail to block development of seizures.[122]

Algorithm 11. Stages and Treatments of AWS	

If patient exhibits or has, within 24 hrs of last drink, 1 or more of following:
 	
• Physiologic: elevated blood pressure, pulse rate, and temperature; sweating
• Neurologic: hand tremors; hyperactive reflexes; agitation; anxiety; seizures
	And clinician rules out:
	• Other pathological processes
	Patient may be in:
	• Stage I AWS
	Then treatment should be:
	• Managing:
	  • Give thiamine (100 mg parenterally for 2-3 days) to avoid onset of WKS
	  • Test for hypoglycemia; if positive, give glucose (<u>always</u> give thiamine first because glucose depletes thiamine reserves)
	  • Maintain hydration and nutrition
	• Sedating:
	  • If needed, give sedative-hypnotic, e.g., oral chlordiazepoxide (100 mg initially; 50 mg 3 hrs later; 25 mg every 3 hrs until patient has been stable for 12 hrs). Note: systolic blood pressure should <u>always</u> be ≥100 before next dose is given
	<u>Note</u>: If patients do not respond to the above sedative-hypnotic doses and require supplemental doses, add magnesium sulfate (2 grams I.M. twice daily for 2-3 days)

If patient exhibits, within 48 hrs of last drink, 1 or more of the following:
 	
• Same as for Stage I, but more severe and/or extensive, <u>plus</u>
• Hallucinations (*See also "alcohol-induced psychotic disorder" in Algorithm 3, Chapter 9.*)
	And clinician rules out:
	• Other pathological processes
	Patient may be in:
	• Stage II AWS
	Then treatment should be:
	• Managing:
	  • Same as for Stage I
	• Sedating:
	  • As long as systolic blood pressure is ≥100, give sedative-hypnotic, e.g., chlordiazepoxide, 100 mg orally each hr; continue until patient is stable, falls asleep, or stops hallucinating. Then, taper dosage as in Stage I

If patient exhibits, within 72 hrs of last drink, 1 or more of the following:
 	
• Same as for Stages I and II, but more severe and/or extensive, <u>plus</u>
• Delirium tremens (*See also "alcohol withdrawal delirium" in Algorithm 3, Chapter 9.*)
	And clinician rules out:
	• Other pathological processes
	Patient may be in:
	• Stage III AWS
	Then treatment should be:
	• Monitoring:
	  • Fluid intake and urinary output; if needed, administer fluids I.V.
	• Testing for and treating as needed:
	  • Hyponatremia, hypocalcemia, hypomagnesemia, hypokalemia, and hypophosphatemia
	• Sedating:
	  • Same as Stage II; however, if sedative-hypnotic must be given parenterally, use medication other than chlordiazepoxide, which is poorly absorbed i.M.

Sedation Monitoring

Oversedation decreases the cough reflex, thereby causing bronchial secretion accumulation and possible pulmonary infection. Undersedation can allow patients' withdrawal to progress to Stages II or III.[148] To avoid over- or undermedicating patients undergoing AWS, clinicians use quantification tools to monitor closely and/or measure the intensity of common withdrawal signs and symptoms. These tools include the Modified Selective Severity Assessment (MSSA)[150] and the Clinical Institute Withdrawal Assessment (CIWA-Ar) scale.[151]

After withdrawal, use of sedatives-hypnotics is not recommended because of the medications' abuse potential and patients' addictive inclinations.[152] However, patients who experience protracted withdrawal, suffering anxiety, depression, and/or insomnia for months after undergoing AWS, even though they remain abstinent, will need treatment for these disorders.

Treatment of Seizures

Seizures can occur during drinking, during AWS, and even following AWS. In alcohol-dependent persons, not all seizures are the direct result of drinking; some may be caused by head trauma, CNS infection, or a preexisting seizure disorder. Therefore, before they are treated, patients with seizures require evaluation tests; e.g., EEG, computerized tomography (CT), and/or magnetic resonance imaging (MRI).[153]

> The majority of alcohol-related seizures are self-limiting; however, some may result in status epilepticus, which can cause neurologic damage or death.

A single seizure presents the risk of arrhythmia, suffocation, and/or injury. The majority of alcohol-related seizures are self-limiting; however, some may result in status epilepticus, which can cause neurologic damage or death.[153] Lechtenberg and Worner[154] report that 83 patients predisposed to seizures not alcohol-related had no seizures during withdrawal when placed on a standard chlordiazepoxide regimen.[117] When a patient is seizure-prone, great caution is required in using antidepressants and phenothiazines, including prochlorperazine (Compazine®).[121]

Use of the antiseizure medication phenytoin (Dilantin®) in treating AWS is controversial. Phenytoin has been associated with serious idiosyncratic reactions; therefore, the American Society of Addiction Medicine (ASAM) Committee on Practice Guidelines has recommended the guidelines shown in Table 21.[153]

The severity of seizures tends to increase progressively in persons who repeatedly undergo alcohol withdrawal. This phenomenon is thought to be analogous to a form of brain sensitization called kindling: small electrical currents, individually too small to produce a seizure, ultimately produce a seizure if applied repeatedly over time. Malcolm et al.[155] report that carbamazepine (Tegretol®) inhibits kindling, and is as effective as oxazepam in treating AWS.[122] However, carbamazepine poses a number of fetal or neonatal risks; if use of the medication is necessary, risks can be minimized by vitamin supplementation (e.g., folate and vitamin K).[143]

Table 21. ASAM Guidelines for Phenytoin Use	
If patient has:	**Then phenytoin is:**
AWS, but no history of seizures	Not recommended
AWS and history of seizures unrelated to alcohol misuse	Recommended, if appropriate for seizure type (otherwise, use other anticonvulsant therapy); also give adequate sedative-hypnotic medication.
AWS and history of alcohol withdrawal seizure	Optional; expert opinion is mixed as to benefit of adding phenytoin to adequate sedative-hypnotic medication
AWS and another disorder which might cause seizures (e.g., head injury, encephalitis)	Optional; no clear consensus among experts
Alcohol withdrawal seizures	Not recommended
Alcohol-related status epilepticus	Recommended; give I.V. phenytoin or other antiseizure therapy

Aversive Medications

Disulfiram (Antabuse®), which causes an unpleasant (aversive) reaction when taken with alcohol, has been a mainstay in treating alcohol dependence; however, this medication has been associated with birth defects and should <u>not</u> be given to pregnant patients.[143] Disulfiram interferes with hepatic metabolism of alcohol, permitting noxious acetaldehyde to accumulate in the blood. (*See Metabolism, Chapter 4.*) Consuming alcohol after taking disulfiram results in rapid heart beat, shortness of breath, headache, nausea, and/or vomiting, thereby discouraging further alcohol consumption.[122]

> Disulfiram is effective for highly motivated, monitored patients taking the medication over an extended period.

The effectiveness of disulfiram is related to the degree to which patients are motivated to stop drinking, and whether they are monitored to ensure medication compliance. Findings in the Veterans' Administration's clinical trial of disulfiram, in the 1980s, were negative because patients failed to take the medication as prescribed. However, Chick et al.[156] recently found disulfiram to be effective for highly motivated, monitored patients taking the medication over an extended period. Short-term use of disulfiram is also effective for patients who have developed some internal control over their cravings, but desire additional protection when in temporary, high-risk situations which involve drinking.

Other research on aversive medications includes:

1. Philips'[157] attempts to develop a long-acting disulfiram formulation which could be injected or incorporated into a time-release surgical implant; as yet, the attempts are unsuccessful and the safety of long-acting disulfiram formulations has not been established

2. Peachey et al.'s[158] controlled study of calcium carbimide, which produces an aversive reaction to alcohol similar to that produced by disulfiram; the study showed that calcium carbimide did not significantly reduce alcohol consumption.

3. Keung's and Vallee's[159] study of daidzin, extracted from the Asian kudzu vine; the compound inhibited alcohol consumption by hamsters but its efficacy in treating alcohol dependence in humans remains to be proven. The idea is not new; in ancient China (600 A.D.), kudzu was used to treat alcohol misuse.[122]

Neuroregulating Medications

Preventing drinking relapses in patients undergoing rehabilitation poses a challenge to clinicians. Clinical trials of various neuroregulating (or anticraving) medications are producing mixed results. These medications, like the neurotransmitters discussed in Chapter 8, bind to and affect the functioning of specific receptors on neurons. Neuroregulating medications act as either agonists, which mimic or enhance neurotransmitters' normal effects on receptors, or antagonists, which block or inhibit those effects.[122]

Table 22 lists neuroregulating medications tested in clinical trials, and their effects on specific receptors. Of these medications, naltrexone and calcium acetylhomotaurinate have been most effective in reinforcing abstinence in alcohol-dependent patients.[122,160]

Table 22. Neuroregulating Medications			
Classes	Generic/Brand Names	Classes	Generic/Brand Names
Dopamine receptor agonist	• Bromocriptine (Parlodel®)	Opioid receptor antagonists	• Naltrexone (ReVia™) • Nalmefene*
Dopamine receptor antagonist	• Tiapride*	Serotonin receptor agonists	• Citalopram* • Fluoxetine (Prozac®) • Zimelidine*
GABA agonist/glutamic acid antagonist	• Calcium acetylhomotaurinate (Acamprosate)*	Serotonin receptor antagonists	• Ondansetron (Zofran®) • Ritanserin* • Sertraline (Zoloft®)

* Not available commercially in the United States

Naltrexone

Alcohol consumption heightens opioid receptor activity, which leads to subjective feelings of craving for more alcohol and an inability to stop drinking. In describing this cycle, many alcohol-dependent persons say: "One drink is too many, and 100 drinks aren't enough."[161]

Naltrexone disrupts the cycle by blocking opioid neurotransmitters from activating their receptors. Clinical trials show that, compared with alcohol-dependent subjects receiving placebos, those taking naltrexone (ReVia®/formerly Trexan®) and undergoing psychotherapy have fewer drinking relapses:

1. Volpicelli et al.[162] — Only 50% of naltrexone-taking subjects who "slipped" (tasted alcohol) during the study relapsed; i.e., naltrexone appeared to stop a slip from becoming a relapse (≥5 drinks on one occasion and/or during the previous week, or having a BAC ≥0.10 g/dL).

2. O'Malley et al.[163] — The type of psychotherapy affected results: compared with placebo-taking subjects, those taking naltrexone and receiving <u>supportive</u> therapy were less likely to experience a slip; subjects taking naltrexone and receiving <u>coping skills</u> therapy slipped as often as placebo-taking subjects but were less likely to relapse.

3. Swift et al.[164] — Compared with subjects taking placebos and drinking a 5-ounce glass of wine, "social" drinkers taking naltrexone and drinking the wine experienced less of a "high" (euphoria); some of the latter also vomited, suggesting that naltrexone may produce an aversive reaction.[161]

In 1994, the Food and Drug Administration (FDA) approved use of naltrexone to treat alcohol dependence only as an adjunct to supportive therapy. Naltrexone is nonaddictive, but higher-than-recommended doses can cause liver toxicity; therefore, the FDA does not recommend its use for patients with active hepatitis or other liver diseases.[152]

Calcium Acetylhomotaurinate

Calcium acetylhomotaurinate (Acamprosate) stimulates the inhibitory effects of gamma-aminobutyric acid (GABA), and antagonizes the excitatory effects of glutamic acid. Therefore, biochemically, the medication may restore the inhibition/excitation balance upset by alcohol consumption.[160]

Whitworth et al.[160] conducted a year-long clinical trial of calcium acetylhomotaurinate on Austrian alcohol-dependent patients; of patients taking the medication and receiving psychosocial therapy, 44% remained abstinent; of patients taking placebos and receiving psychosocial therapy, only 19% remained abstinent. Therefore, the researchers believe that calcium acetylhomotaurinate compares favorably with naltrexone in reducing drinking relapse rate.

The Next Step

It is unlikely that any single medication will be effective for all alcohol-dependent patients. Further research is needed to identify "responder" subpopulations (whose characteristics predispose them to have the most success with a certain medication), so that each group can receive the appropriate pharmacological interventions.[161]

Chapter Summary

1. The majority of patients undergoing AWS will respond to reassurance and supportive measures, with no need of sedatives-hypnotics.

2. Clinicians must know patients' BACs before giving them sedatives-hypnotics; using these medications to treat patients with high BACs can provoke a synergistic reaction with alcohol, resulting in hypotension, shock, or coma.

3. To avoid over- or undermedicating patients undergoing AWS, clinicians use quantification tools such as the Modified Selective Severity Assessment (MSSA) and the Clinical Institute Withdrawal Assessment (CIWA-Ar) scale.

4. Before they are treated, patients with seizures require evaluation tests; e.g., EEG, CT, and/or MRI.

5. Use of the anticonvulsant phenytoin (Dilantin®) in treating AWS is controversial; American Society of Addiction Medicine (ASAM) guidelines for phenytoin use should be followed.

6. Disulfiram, which causes an aversive reaction when taken with alcohol, has been a mainstay of alcohol-dependence treatment; however, because it has been associated with birth defects, disulfiram should not be given to pregnant patients.

7. Among neuroregulating (or anticraving) medications undergoing clinical trials, naltrexone (ReVia™) and calcium acetylhomotaurinate (Acamprosate) have been most effective in reinforcing abstinence in alcohol-dependent patients.

Chapter 13 Recovery

Participation in Alcoholics Anonymous (A.A.) is the keystone of patients' recovery from alcohol misuse. Recovery can also involve use of pharmacotherapy, supplemented by cognitive-behavioral therapy, to prevent relapse. Patients increase their chances of maintaining sobriety when, after medical detoxification, their post-AWS treatment plan matches their particular characteristics (e.g., treatment and demographic history, personality, psychosocial functioning, psychiatric disorders, social support).[165]

"Justifications" for Relapse

Ludwig[166] has found that some abstinent, alcohol-dependent patients put themselves in situations conducive to resumption of drinking. Such behavior occurs when, e.g., recovering drinkers:

1. Attend parties, "accidentally" pick up someone else's drink, and sip on it
2. Buy alcohol-containing cough medicine or mouthwash (*For alcohol content of mouthwashes, see Appendix B.)*
3. Drink the sacramental wine when receiving communion
4. Drop by their once-favorite bar <u>just</u> to see their friends.[166]

Ludwig also found that nine overlapping thought/attitude patterns caused many patients to relapse:

1. Escape from unpleasantness — *I will feel numb and be at peace.*
2. Improved self image — *I will feel good about myself, even when I'm alone.*
3. No control — *I'm too weak-willed to give up alcohol, so why bother?*
4. Relaxation — *I desperately need a couple of drinks after driving home for 2 hours in all that traffic.*
5. Romance — *This awful lonely feeling will go away if I have a few drinks and fantasize about sex.*
6. Self-control — *I'll have just one beer; I've got things under control now.*

7. Sensual pleasure — *Oh, how I long for the warm feeling of a shot of bourbon trickling down into my stomach.*
8. Social lubricant — *I'm lots of fun at parties after I've had a few glasses of wine.*
9. To hell with it — *Nothing really matters in my life, so why not drink?*[166]

Twelve-Step Programs

Twelve-step programs include Alcoholics Anonymous, which helps persons who have misused alcohol to abstain, and Al-Anon, Alateen, and Adult Children of Alcoholics which help family members to recover from the pain and stress of living with an alcohol-dependent person.

Alcoholics Anonymous

Alcoholics Anonymous (A.A.) is the most popular recovery support group for persons who desire to stop drinking. Self-help through A.A. is the only addiction treatment many people receive.[167]

Table 23. A.A. Statistics (Estimated, 1996)
• U.S. membership — 1.2 million
• Worldwide membership — 1.8 million
• Groups in U.S. — 51,000
• Groups worldwide — 90,000
• Countries with A.A. groups — 140

A.A. was founded in 1935 by two alcohol-dependent persons: stockbroker William Griffith Wilson (known as Bill W.) and physician Robert H. Smith (known as Dr. Bob). One day, Bill W., who had been abstinent for 5 months, felt a tremendous need to drink, so he arranged to talk with Dr. Bob about their common problem. Bill W. discovered that this interaction abated his drinking compulsion for that day. Subsequently, the two men arranged meetings between other alcoholics, and formulated the basic A.A. philosophy. By 1946, when A.A.'s Twelve Traditions were first drafted, membership numbered about 15,000; from a modest beginning, A.A. membership and distribution have mushroomed (*see Table 23*), despite a high dropout rate.[10,168]

Clinicians who familiarize themselves with A.A.'s Twelve Steps and Twelve Traditions (*see Table 24*) realize A.A. can be a valuable resource for many addicted patients. Clinicians can also learn about A.A. by accompanying a patient, or going alone, to an open meeting, as well as by reading *Alcoholics Anonymous* (or, as members call it, the "Big Book"); they are then prepared to respond to patients' objections to attending the meetings, e.g.:

1. "Then everybody will know I'm a drunk" — *A.A., by name, is an anonymous group; no member has the right to reveal what is said at a meeting, or who said it.*

Table 24. The Twelve Steps and Traditions of A.A.*	
The Twelve Steps	**The Twelve Traditions**
1. We admitted we were powerless over alcohol—that our lives had become unmanageable.	1. Our common welfare should come first; personal recovery depends upon A.A. unity.
2. Came to believe that a Power greater than ourselves could restore us to sanity	2. For our group purpose, there is but one ultimate authority— a loving God as He may express Himself in our group conscience. Our leaders are but trusted servants; they do not govern.
3. Made a decision to turn our will and our lives over to the care of God *as we understood Him*	3. The only requirement for A.A. membership is a desire to stop drinking.
4. Made a searching and fearless moral inventory of ourselves	4. Each group should be autonomous except in matters affecting other groups or A.A. as a whole.
5. Admitted to God, to ourselves and to another human being the exact nature of our wrongs	5. Each group has but one primary purpose—to carry its message to the alcoholic who still suffers.
6. Were entirely ready to have God remove all these defects of character	6. An A.A. group ought never endorse, finance, or lend the A.A. name to any related facility or outside enterprise, lest problems of money, property, and prestige divert us from our primary purpose.
7. Humbly asked Him to remove our shortcomings	7. Every A.A. group ought to be fully self-supporting, declining outside contributions.
8. Made a list of all persons we had harmed and became willing to make amends to them all	8. Alcoholics Anonymous should remain forever non-professional, but our service centers may employ special workers.
9. Made direct amends to such people wherever possible, except when to do so would injure them or others	9. A.A., as such, ought never be organized; but we may create service boards or committees directly responsible to those they serve.
10. Continued to take personal inventory and when we were wrong promptly admitted it	10. Alcoholics Anonymous has no opinion on outside issues; hence the A.A. name ought never be drawn into public controversy.
11. Sought through prayer and meditation to improve our conscious contact with God *as we understood Him,* praying only for knowledge of His will for us and the power to carry that out	11. Our public relations policy is based on attraction rather than promotion; we need always maintain personal anonymity at the level of press, radio, and films.
12. Having had a spiritual awakening as the result of these steps, we tried to carry this message to alcoholics, and to practice these principles in all our affairs.	12. Anonymity is the spiritual foundation of all our traditions, ever reminding us to place principles before personalities.

* The Twelve Steps and Twelve Traditions are reprinted with permission of Alcoholics Anonymous World Services, Inc. Permission to reprint the Twelve Steps and Twelve Traditions does not mean that A.A. has reviewed or approved the contents of this publication, nor that A.A. agrees with the views expressed herein. A.A. is a program of recovery from alcoholism only—use of the Twelve Steps and Twelve Traditions in connection with programs and activities which are patterned after A.A., but which address other problems, or in any other non-A.A. context, does not imply otherwise.

2. "The judge suspended my driver's license; I can't go anywhere" — *A.A. will make arrangements for you, if you ask.*
3. "I'm not going to stand up in front of people and tell them my problems" — *If you feel uncomfortable about talking in front of the group, simply say you 'pass' on the opportunity; the group will respect your wishes.*

4. "I'm never going to be able to stop drinking" — *A.A. asks only that you have a desire to stop drinking; I know you have that desire.*
5. "You know my allergies act up when I'm in a smoky room" — *We will find a non-smoking group, or one that divides its meetings into smoking and non-smoking sections.*
6. "I don't need all that religion" — *Please understand that A.A. is a spiritual program, not a religion; members use the slogan "Let go and let God" to help them realize there is a higher power ("God, as we understand Him") to help them, if they can just "let go" of their frustrations. Members in difficult situations also rely on The Serenity Prayer.*[168,169]

> ***The Serenity Prayer***: *God grant me the serenity to accept the things I cannot change, the courage to change the things that I can, and the wisdom to know the difference.*

Clinicians should help each patient choose an A.A. "home group" (which serves as an extended family) and a same-sex sponsor who has been continuously sober for about 1 year. A.A. newcomers often talk with their sponsors several times a day, whenever they think about drinking or are frustrated by problems. This allows sponsors to "keep sobriety by giving it away," just as Bill W. found he could stay sober by sharing his story with other drinkers trying to stay sober.[10,169]

All patients should be cautioned that A.A. members may give them inappropriate advice about stopping use of medications (even though A.A. policy encourages members to <u>comply</u> with their physicians' recommendations). Young female patients should be cautioned that "Thirteenth Stepping" (older men taking advantage of the trustful atmosphere of A.A. meetings to approach newly recovering young women) has, on occasion, been reported.[169,170]

> Clinicians must periodically check patients for warning signs of an impending relapse.

Analyses of five surveys during 1977 to 1989 suggest that about half of persons joining A.A. drop out within 3 months. A.A. does not have any formal control over its members; therefore, clinicians must periodically check patients for warning signs of an impending relapse (e.g., patients who are unwilling to discuss their A.A. experiences may have stopped attending meetings and may request medications to relieve their anxiety).[168,169]

Few patients who <u>regularly</u> attend A.A. meetings relapse; therefore, when patients report they feel uncomfortable at their particular A.A. home group, clinicians should determine if a special interest group is available in their locale. Most large metropolitan areas have special A.A. meetings for women, adolescents, elders, homosexuals, ethnic groups, racial groups, health care workers, lawyers, and clergy.[168,169]

Family Support Groups

While Bill W. was occupied with A.A. meetings, his wife, Lois, became aware of her own negative emotions and recurring urge to derail Bill's emerging sobriety; therefore, she formed a support group for spouses. This eventually led to development of Al-Anon, which modified A.A.'s Twelve Steps and Twelve Traditions slightly; its groups could then provide family members with support and nurturing, and, eventually, recovery from the ripple effect of living with an alcohol-dependent person.[10] Alateen, started by a California teenager in 1957, follows Al-Anon steps and traditions; each Alateen group has an active Al-Anon member as a sponsor.

Adult Children of Alcoholics (ACOA), which developed during the 1980s, provides support for these family members. Clinicians should try to identify them and intervene. Woititz[171] reports that such patients exhibit common characteristics, including severe self-judging, impulsivity, dishonesty, denial, suppressed feelings, and secretiveness.

Cognitive-Behavioral Therapy

Cognitive-behavioral approaches include relapse prevention training, coping skills training, and family therapeutic interventions; these teach patients the skills they need to confront or avoid everyday situations which may lead to drinking. Patients first identify their particular drinking antecedents (e.g., anger, depression, peer influence) and positive drinking consequences (e.g., reduced anxiety, increased self-esteem), then identify ways to alter these learned behaviors.[172]

Relapse Prevention Training

This type of training focuses on interrupting the relapse process and identifying behaviors which should be strengthened to maintain long-term sobriety. Marlatt[173] believes recovering drinkers respond to high-risk situations either by:

1. Choosing and making use of appropriate coping responses — they feel a sense of mastery and an ability to deal with the situation, decreasing the likelihood of a relapse, or
2. Not using adequate coping responses — they feel helpless, expect that a drink would help in the situation, start drinking, and experience a syndrome Marlatt calls the "abstinence violation effect" (patients contrast their previous perceptions of being in

recovery with the current reality of renewed drinking; this causes feelings of conflict, guilt, self-blame, and loss of control, increasing the probability of a full-blown relapse).[172]

Relapse prevention therapists use the following interventions to help patients avoid high-risk situations:

1. Modifying patients' lifestyles by strengthening behaviors which are incompatible with drinking
2. Providing decision-making and self-control training which enables patients to make appropriate choices
3. Establishing a balance between the time clients spend fulfilling responsibilities and the time they spend on pleasurable activities.[172,174]

Coping Skills Training

Monti et al.[175] recommend that the following intrapersonal and interpersonal skills be included in a coping skills program:

1. Intrapersonal skills — managing cravings, anger, and negative thinking; decision-making; emergency planning; problem-solving; relaxation training
2. Interpersonal skills — Resisting social pressures to drink; learning to start conversations, be assertive, say "no" to overburdening requests, and communicate feelings; learning to give and receive compliments and criticism.[172]

Therapists should encourage patients to fill their leisure time previously used for drinking; patients should sample various leisure activities to find those which (1) they enjoy, (2) are incompatible with drinking, and (3) could be used as rewards for specific accomplishments on the road to sobriety.[172]

Family Therapeutic Interventions

Family members generally require education about alcohol misuse, as well as opportunities to discuss the impact that a loved one's alcohol dependence is having on their lives. Therapeutic interventions for family members include:

1. Training in communication skills, conflict resolution, and problem-solving
2. Breaking the cycle of criticism and recriminations
3. Providing praise for positive changes
4. Discovering shared leisure activities.[172]

To help structure these new interactions, therapists can assist family members to formulate behavior contracts which specify each person's role.[172] Galanter[176] stresses, e.g., that spouses must be involved in appropriate ways: they must not be placed in the position of pressing the patient to comply with treatment. For patients taking disulfiram, spouses should not actively remind patient-spouses to take the drug; they should merely notify therapists if they do not see their patient-spouses ingesting the medication on schedule. This action shifts compliance management to the therapists.

Mandated Treatment

In recent decades, institutions, such as courts and workplaces, have been mandating referrals for alcohol misuse treatment with increasing frequency. Criminal justice system referrals typically result from charges of public drunkenness, crimes such as domestic violence in which alcohol use is suspected to have been a contributing factor, and alcohol-specific offenses such as driving under the influence (DUI). Studies of the effectiveness of mandated treatment for DUI offenders show that, on average, treated offenders repeat their offenses 8% to 9% less often than untreated offenders.[177] Wells-Parker[177] recommends that, to enhance general traffic safety, licensing sanctions should be combined with DUI offender rehabilitation programs.

Chapter Summary

1. The keystone of patients' recovery from alcohol misuse is participation in Alcoholics Anonymous (A.A.).

2. Some recovering drinkers put themselves in situations conducive to resumption of drinking.

3. By familiarizing themselves with A.A., clinicians can respond to patients' objections to attending the meetings.

4. Support groups for family members living with an alcohol-dependent person include Al-Anon, Alateen, and ACOA.

5. Cognitive-behavioral therapy includes training in relapse prevention and coping skills, and family interventions.

6. Relapse prevention training focuses on interrupting the relapse process and identifying and strengthening positive behaviors.

7. Family members must formulate behavior contracts which clearly specify each person's role.

Progress Test G (Chapters 12 & 13)

1. Benzer's suggested rule of thumb is "to withhold medications for treating AWS symptoms while patients have BACs of _____."

2. To avoid over- or undermedicating patients undergoing AWS, clinicians use _____ tools.

3. Use of the anticonvulsant phenytoin in treating AWS is _____, because the drug has been associated with serious idiosyncratic reactions.

4. Disulfiram has been found to be effective for highly motivated, _____ patients taking the medication over an extended period.

5. Naltrexone blocks _____ neurotransmitters from activating their receptors.

6. Clinicians who familiarize themselves with A.A's Twelve _____ and Twelve _____, as well as other A.A. practices, are prepared to respond to patients' objections to attend the meetings.

7. Recovering drinkers not using adequate coping responses may experience the _____ _____ effect.

8. Coping skills therapy involves _____ and _____ skills.

9. On average, treated DUI offenders repeat their offenses _____ ____ _____ less often than untreated offenders.

Definitions, Abbreviations, & Acronyms

Acetate — an acetic acid salt.

Acetic acid — an aqueous solution of CH_3COOH; a 4% to 6% solution is vinegar; also a product of alcohol metabolism.

Acinar cell — any cell lining an acinus (or small sac-like structure); in particular, a proenzyme-secreting cell of a pancreatic acinus.

Addiction — physical and psychologic dependence, including tolerance of a drug, withdrawal symptoms when use is stopped, and persistent relapses following reversal of physical dependence.

Agoraphobia — abnormal fear of or anxiety about being in open or public places or situations.

Alcohol — a hydroxyl group compound, i.e., an oxygen and a hydrogen molecule (—OH) bonded to a carbon molecule.

Alcohol abuse — a category of alcohol misuse; despite persistent or recurrent interpersonal or social problems, drinkers continue to drink to excess.

Alcohol dehydrogenase — an enzyme in human tissue; it oxidizes alcohols to other compounds known as aldehydes and ketones; however, it also acts as a catalyst, reducing aldehydes and ketones to alcohols.

Alcohol dependence — a category of alcohol misuse; drinkers have developed clinically significant impairment or distress, manifesting particular symptoms, e.g., tolerance, withdrawal, impaired control, preoccupation with drinking, and drinking despite problems.

Alcoholic myopathy — a muscle disorder characterized by proximal limb weakness and presence of myoglobulin in the urine.

Alcoholism — *See Alcohol dependence.*

Alcohol misuse — any excessive or clearly destructive drinking. *For categories of misuse, see Alcohol abuse; Alcohol dependence; Hazardous drinking; Mild alcohol problems.*

Alcohol withdrawal syndrome — the onset of certain signs and symptoms following the abrupt discontinuation of, or rapid decrease in, consumption of alcohol.

Alkaline phosphatase — an enzyme involved in bone mineralization.

Allele — one of two or more versions of the same gene occupying the same position on a particular chromosome.

Amblyopia — impaired vision without detectable, organic, optic lesions.

Ammonia — a neurotoxic chemical compound formed in the body, primarily as a product of protein metabolism; in the liver, ammonia is transformed into less toxic urea, which is excreted in urine.

Amnesia — memory loss. *See Anterograde amnesia; Blackout; Retrograde amnesia.*

Angular cheilitis — inflammation and cracks at the corners of the lips.

Anorexia — loss of appetite and inability to eat.

Anterograde amnesia — the inability, after onset of amnesia, to learn and form new memories.

Antipsychotic — a medication used to treat certain mental and emotional conditions, including psychosis.

AOD — alcohol and other drug abuse.

Arcus senilis — an opaque, white ring around the cornea periphery.

Arrhythmia — irregular or abnormal rhythm of the heart beat.

ASAM — American Society of Addiction Medicine.

Ascites — accumulation of fluid in the abdominal cavity.

Aspirin — acetylsalicylic acid; a medication used to treat pain, fever, and inflammation.

Asterixis — also called flapping tremor. A neurologic disorder characterized by involuntary jerking movements, especially of the hands; it is frequently demonstrated by patients in hepatic coma.

Asymptomatic — without symptoms. (*See Symptom.*)

Ataxia — defective voluntary muscular coordination.

Atrial fibrillation — rapid, incomplete contractions of the atria (upper chambers of heart).

Atrophy — a wasting away, deterioration, or shrinkage, especially of a body part or organ.

AWS — alcohol withdrawal syndrome.

BAC — blood alcohol concentration.

Beta-blocker — a medication (e.g., propranolol) which blocks activity of epinephrine at ß-adrenergic receptors.

Bilirubin — a yellowish-orange pigment in bile; an excess of bilirubin in the blood may cause jaundice.

Binge drinking — consumption of ≥5 drinks at one sitting.

Blackout — a type of amnesia occasionally associated with rapidly increasing BAC.

Blood alcohol concentration — the weight of alcohol in a specific volume of blood, expressed in g/dL. (*See Table 3 for equivalencies.*)

Blood plasma — the pale yellow liquid in which red and white blood cells and platelets are suspended.

Blood serum — the clear liquid which separates from blood when it clots completely.

Bone marrow — the red or yellow, soft, fatty tissue found in bone cavities. Red bone marrow is blood-producing tissue, gradually replaced in some bones, as the body ages, by less active yellow marrow.

BrAC — breath-alcohol concentration.

Bradykinesia — abnormal slowness; sluggish mental and physical responses. *See Parkinson's disease.*

Bruxism — grinding of the teeth.

Carbohydrate-deficient transferrin — an abnormal variant of transferrin; found in higher amounts in persons abusing alcohol. (*See Transferrin.*)

Cardiomyopathy — disease of the heart muscle.

Centrocecal scotoma — a horizontal, oval defect in the field of vision, involving the blind spot and the fixation point.

Cholestasis — suppression or stoppage of bile flow.

Chronic drinking — consumption of alcohol, usually on a daily basis and in large quantities, over a long period.

Cimetidine — a medication used to inhibit gastric secretion.

CNS — central nervous system; includes the brain and spinal cord.

Cognition (adj. cognitive) — the mental process of knowing, including such things as awareness, perception, judgment, and reasoning.

Collagen — the fibrous protein constituent of connective tissue.

Coma — deep unconsciousness, often prolonged; usually resulting from injury, disease, or drugs.

Confabulation — unconscious fabrication of stories to fill in memory gaps; characteristic of patients with Korsakoff psychosis or other organic amnestic disorders.

Congener — a secondary product of fermentation, e.g., methanol, butanol, histamine, tannic acid, and fusel oil.

Consciousness — a state of awareness of one's environment and existence, including thoughts and sensations. (*See also Unconsciousness.*)

Convulsion — a seizure symptom; characterized by twitching and jerking of the limbs.

Cortisol — a hormone secreted by the adrenal cortex.

CSAT — Center for Substance Abuse Treatment.

Cytoplasm — the region within a cell which lies outside the nucleus.

Cytosol (adj. cytosolic) — the fluid portion of the cytoplasm.

Delirium tremens (DTs) — a state of confusion accompanied by trembling and vivid hallucinations.

Delusion — a strongly held false belief or opinion about external reality, despite invalidating proof or evidence.

Dementia — a general loss of intellectual abilities, including memory, judgment, and abstract thinking.

Dendrite — one of many branched appendages of a neuron which receive incoming signals and transmit them to the cell body. (*See Fig. 9.*)

Depersonalization — sense of being detached from oneself.

Depression, mental — a condition marked by deep sadness and lack of any pleasurable interest in life.

Derealization — feeling of unreality

Detoxification — the process of safely freeing a drug user from an addictive drug (e.g., alcohol).

Diabetes mellitus — a chronic syndrome causing impaired metabolism of proteins, fats, and carbohydrates; the result of insufficient insulin secretion.

Disorientation — confusion about direction, location, time, and/or identity.

Diuretic — an agent which promotes urine excretion.

Drinker — a person who drinks alcohol. *See Chronic drinker.*

Drinking — consumption of alcohol. *See Binge drinking; Chronic drinking; Heavy drinking; Moderate drinking, Social drinking; Very heavy drinking.*

DSM-IV — *Diagnostic and Statistical Manual of Mental Disorders,* 4th edition, published by the American Psychiatric Association.

Dupuytren's contracture — palmar fascia contracture; the ring and little fingers are bent into the palm and can no longer be extended.

Dysarthria — impaired ability to articulate due to emotional stress, brain injury, paralysis, or incoordination of the muscles used for speaking.

Dysesthesia — an unpleasant, abnormal sensation (e.g., burning, numbness, tingling, prickling, or cutting pain) produced by normal stimuli. (*See also Paresthesia*)

Dysphagia — swallowing difficulty or inability.

Dysrhythmia — rhythm disturbance; e.g., ventricular dysrhythmia of the heart.

Edema — swelling, caused by excessive accumulation of fluid in tissues.

Electrocardiogram (EKG) — a graphic tracing of electrical potential variations of the heart muscle and cardiac nerves

Electroencephalogram (EEG) — a recording of the brain's electrical activity; variations in EEG patterns correlate well with activity and conditions in the brain.

Encephalitis — inflammation of the brain.

Encephalopathy — any degenerative brain disease.

Endoscope (adj. endoscopic) — an instrument used to examine the inside of large body organs.

Enzyme — any highly specialized protein which catalyzes a specific chemical reaction.

Epidural hematoma — an accumulation of blood, sometimes under pressure, upon the dura mater, the outermost covering of the brain and spinal cord.

Erythema — redness of the skin

Esophagitis — inflammation of the esophagus.

Ethanol (also ethyl alcohol, CH_3CH_2OH) — an alcohol which occurs naturally as a product of sugar fermentation and can be consumed as a beverage, in <u>limited</u> amounts, without ill effects.

Florid vascular spider — *see Vascular spider.*

Folate — a folic acid ester or salt.

Folliculitis — inflammation of hair follicles.

Furfural — a liquid aldehyde; in alcoholic beverages, a congener released by some wooden casks.

Gamma-glutamyl transferase (GGT) — an enzyme involved in protein metabolism; long-term excessive alcohol consumption causes GGT to be released from the liver into the bloodstream.

Gastric — pertaining to, affecting, or originating in the stomach.

Gastritis — inflammation of the stomach.

Gastroesophageal reflux — the return of stomach contents into the esophagus.

g/dL — grams per deciliter.

Gene — a sequence of nucleotides (i.e., the basic molecular units of deoxyribonucleic acid—DNA) which, when translated by mechanisms in a cell, encode a protein. Genes are inherited and determine the specific characteristics of all living things.

Glossitis — inflammation of the tongue.

Glutathione — a compound comprising glutamate, glycine, and cysteine.

Gout — an inflammatory, arthritic condition characterized by uric acid crystal deposits in joint spaces.

Grand mal seizure — a sudden loss of consciousness, followed by violent convulsions. *See Convulsion; Seizure.*

Greater than — >; greater than or equal to — ≥.

H_2 — one of two types of cellular receptor sites for histamine; H_2 receptors promote gastric acid secretion and mediate heart-rate acceleration.

Hallucination — a seemingly real sensory perception that occurs despite absence of stimulation of the relevant sensory organ.

Hazardous drinking — a category of alcohol misuse; drinkers do not yet have alcohol-related problems, but occasionally increase their risk when they drink, then engage in certain activities.

Heavy drinking — consumption of ≥2 drinks per day, or ≥14 drinks per week.

Hemorrhagic stroke — hemorrhage into the brain, usually accompanied by sudden loss of consciousness, followed by paralysis.

Hepatitis — an inflammation of the liver, caused by viruses or other toxins.

Hepatocellular — pertaining to, or affecting, liver cells.

High-density lipoprotein (HDL) — a type of blood lipoprotein particle with a density of 1.063-1.21 g/mL.

Homeostasis — the maintenance of the body's relatively steady internal environment. *See Stress response.*

Hyperglycemia — higher-than-normal concentration of blood glucose; caused by impaired insulin secretion.

Hypersomnia — difficulty in staying awake.

Hypertension — abnormally high blood pressure. *See Portal hypertension; Pulmonary hypertension.*

Hyperuricemia — an abnormal concentration of uric acid or urates in the blood.

Hypocalcemia — abnormally low concentration of blood calcium.

Hypoglycemia (adj. hypoglycemic) — abnormally low concentration of blood glucose.

Hypokalemia — abnormally low concentration of blood potassium.

Hypomagnesemia — abnormally low concentration of blood plasma magnesium.

Hyponatremia — decreased concentration of blood sodium.

Hypophosphatemia — abnormally low concentration of blood phosphates.

ICD-10 — *International Classification of Diseases,* 10th edition, published by the World Health Organization.

I.M. — by intramuscular injection.

I.U. — international units.

I.V. — by intravenous injection.

Infarction — an area of dying tissue caused by an obstructed blood supply.

Insomnia — difficulty in falling or staying asleep or poor sleep quality.

Intoxication — dysfunctional physiologic and psychologic changes caused by consumption of a psychoactive substance (e.g., alcohol).

Ischemic stroke — diminished blood supply to the brain, usually accompanied by sudden loss of consciousness, followed by paralysis.

JAMA — *Journal of the American Medical Association.*

Kcal — kilocalorie.

Kernicterus (also bilirubin encephalopathy) — a condition associated with abnormally high bilirubin levels in the blood; characterized by severe, destructive neural changes.

Less than — <; less than or equal to — ≤.

Leukocytosis — an abnormal number of white blood cells; a transient condition.

Lipid — a fat or fat-like substance not soluble in water.

Macrocytosis — a condition in which red blood cells are abnormally large.

Magnetic resonance imaging (MRI) — an imaging technique which provides high-quality, three-dimensional images of organs and structures inside the body, without using X-rays or other radiation.

Mallory-Weiss tear — a rupture in the opening from the esophagus to the stomach.

Mania (adj. manic) — abnormally and persistently elevated, expansive, or irritable mood or behavior.

Marker — a laboratory-derived sign of excessive and harmful alcohol consumption.

Mean corpuscular volume (MCV) — a measure of red blood cell volume, expressed in cubic micrometers.

Methanol (also methyl alcohol or wood alcohol; CH_3OH) — a poisonous alcohol which, if ingested, can cause blindness; methanol is a very minor ingredient of some hard liquors. (*See Chapter 4.*)

Mild alcohol problems — a category of alcohol misuse; drinkers' lives are negatively affected; however, the problems are not as serious as those which accompany alcohol abuse. *See Alcohol abuse.*

Mitochondrion — a tiny, membrane-enclosed cell structure; produces energy that can be used by the cell.

Moderate drinking — for men, consumption of a maximum of two drinks per day; for women, a maximum of 1 drink per day.

Mood — a pervasive, sustained emotion which changes one's perception of the world; "abnormal" moods include depression (e.g., sadness), elevation (e.g., euphoria or elation), expansiveness (e.g., unrestrained expression of feelings), or irritability (e.g., easily annoyed).

Mood disorder — a depressive and/or manic ailment.

Mucosa — mucous membrane.

Multi-infarct dementia — a general loss of intellectual abilities with a stepwise deteriorating course, due to a series of small strokes.

Murmur — an abnormal, short, periodic sound of cardiovascular origin.

Myelin — a white, fatty substance enclosing various nerve axons and fibers; it facilitates conduction of nerve impulses.

Myocardium (adj., myocardial) — the middle, thickest muscle layer of the heart wall.

Myopathy — disease of striated muscle.

NCADI — National Clearinghouse on Alcohol and Drug Information.

Necrosis — cell death, caused by the progressive degradation of enzyme action.

Neonatal — pertaining to the first 4 weeks of an infant's life.

Neuron — a cell in the brain, spinal cord, or other parts of the body which conducts electrical impulses.

Neurotoxic — capable of damaging or destroying nerve tissue.

Neurotransmitter — a neuron-released chemical substance ("chemical messenger") which crosses a synapse to bind to a receptor on an adjacent neuron; neurotransmitters include acetylcholine, dopamine, gamma-aminobutyric acid, glutamic acid, norepinephrine, opioid, and serotonin.

Neurotransmitter receptor — a protein, located on the outer surface of a neuron, which binds with a specific neurotransmitter; this either triggers electrical impulses in the receiving neuron, or reduces the neuron's sensitivity to other incoming messages.

NIAAA — National Institute on Alcohol Abuse and Alcoholism.

NIDA — National Institute on Drug Abuse.

NIH — National Institutes of Health.

NLAES — National Longitudinal Alcohol Epidemiologic Survey.

Nystagmus — involuntary, rapid eyeball movement.

Opioid — (1) a medication or drug containing, or derived from, opium; (2) a medication or drug with opioid-like effects but not derived from opium; (3) a neurotransmitter.

Oropharynx (adj. oropharyngeal) — the portion of the pharynx lying between the soft palate and the upper edge of the epiglottis

Osteomyelitis — inflammation of bone caused by pathogens.

Osteoporosis — a reduction in bone mass.

Overdose — inadvertent or deliberate consumption of a larger dose of a substance than is habitually taken, resulting in serious toxicity or death.

Palpitation — an abnormally rapid fluttering or throbbing of the heart.

Pancreatitis — inflammation of the pancreas.

Panic attack — sudden, intense feelings of alarm, fear, or terror.

Paresthesia — a skin sensation, e.g., burning, prickling, tingling, or itching, with no apparent physical cause. (*See also Dysesthesia.*)

Parkinson's disease — a slowly progressive neurologic disorder, characterized by rigidity, tremor, postural instability, and bradykinesia. *See Bradykinesia.*

Parotid gland — one of a pair of salivary glands situated on the sides of the face below and in front of the ears.

Peptic ulcer — erosion of the mucosa along the lesser curvature of the stomach, at the lower end of the esophagus, or in the duodenum (first part of small intestine).

Per capita consumption — average amount of alcohol imbibed annually by each person, ≥14 years of age, in the United States; such statistics do not mean that all residents consumed alcohol or that drinkers consumed it in equal amounts.

Periodontitis — inflammation of the tissue around the teeth.

Peripheral neuropathy — diseases and disorders affecting the nerves that fan out from the CNS to the muscles, skin, internal organs, and glands.

Placebo — an innocuous or inert substance used as a control in clinical trials of a new medication.

Platelet — a small, disk-shaped body in blood; plays an important role in blood clotting.

Portal hypertension — abnormally increased blood pressure in the portal vein of the liver.

Postural hypotension — a decrease in blood pressure, upon standing up.

Prolactin — a hormone produced by the anterior pituitary gland.

Proteolysis (adj. proteolytic) — the hydrolysis (or splitting) of proteins or peptides, forming smaller products; some enzymes promote proteolysis.

Psoriasis — a chronic skin disease, characterized by erythematous papules forming plaques with distinct borders.

Psychoactive medication — any drug that directly affects the functioning of the mind or the brain.

Psychomotor agitation — excessive, usually repetitious, physical behavior accompanying emotional strain; e.g., pacing, fidgeting.

Psychosis (adj. psychotic) — historically, this term has been applied to many disorders; in general, it can be defined as clinically significant impairment of mental functioning which prevents a sufferer from meeting the ordinary demands of life.

Pulmonary hypertension — abnormally increased blood pressure within the circulation of the lungs.

Purine — an end product of nucleoprotein digestion, which then breaks down into uric acid. *See Uric acid.*

Pylorospasm — spasmodic contraction of the opening (pyloric orifice) between the stomach and duodenum.

Receptor — *see Neurotransmitter receptor.*

Relapse — resumption of alcohol or other drug use by an individual who has been abstinent for a significant time following detoxification.

Reticulocytosis — a higher-than-normal number of immature red blood cells.

Retrograde amnesia — loss of memories stored prior to the onset of amnesia.

Rhinophyma — a bulbous red nose caused by untreated rosacea. (*See Rosacea.*)

Rosacea — a facial skin disease; characterized by papules, pustules, and hyperplasia of soft tissues of the nose. (*See Rhinophyma.*)

SAMHSA — Substance Abuse and Mental Health Services Administration.

Sclerotherapy — injecting sclerosing (hardening) solutions to treat esophageal varices, hemorrhoids, or varicose veins.

Scotoma — a visual field area of lost or depressed vision, surrounded by an area of normal or less depressed vision. (*See Centrocecal scotoma.*)

Seborrheic dermatitis — an inflammatory skin disease, characterized by lesions covered with yellow or brown-gray scales.

Sedative-hypnotic — a medication to quiet or induce sleep; used to treat excessive nervousness, restlessness, or insomnia.

Seizure — a sudden episode of uncontrolled electrical activity in the brain. *See also Grand mal seizure; Convulsion.*

Sign — objective indication of disease, especially abnormal, observable physical, radiologic, and laboratory evidence.

Sixth nerve palsy — an inward deviation of the eye.

Sobriety — continuous abstinence from alcohol and other drugs.

Social drinking — occasional light consumption of alcohol in company with others.

Status epilepticus — a series of convulsions, rapidly repeated and with no periods of consciousness between them.

Stomatitis — inflammation of oral mucosa.

Stress response — a reaction to a threat to homeostasis; it involves the central nervous, adrenal, and cardiovascular systems. First, the hypothalamus secretes corticotropin releasing factor, which triggers the pituitary gland to release adrenocorticotropin hormone; this, in turn, triggers the adrenal gland to secrete glucocorticoid hormones. *See Homeostasis.*

Stressor — any event or change in a person's life which may be associated with the onset or exacerbation of a psychologic response. (*See Stress response.*)

Sublingual — under the tongue.

Symptom — a subjective indication of disease, especially a patient's report of an abnormal physical or emotional condition.

Synapse — the microscopic gap between any two neurons.

Synergism (adj. synergistic) — a harmonious action of two drugs, producing an effect which is greater than the total effects of each drug alone, or one that neither drug could produce alone.

Tachycardia — abnormally rapid heart beat; in adults, over 100 beats per minute.

Teratogen — any substance which can cause physical defects in a developing embryo.

Thiamine — Vitamin B_1; essential for growth and required for normal brain functioning.

Third-party payer — payer other than the patient for services; e.g., private insurance companies and public payers such as Medicare and Medicaid.

Thrombocytopenia — a diminished blood platelet count.

Tolerance — the need for higher and higher doses of a drug to achieve the same effects.

Transferrin — a blood serum beta globulin which combines with and transports iron.

Trauma — an injury caused by an extrinsic agent, or a disordered psychologic state resulting from physical injury or stress.

Tremor — an involuntary and rhythmic movement in the muscles of parts of the body, most often the hands, feet, jaw, tongue, or head.

Triglyceride — a combination of cholesterol and fatty acids; the principal component of oils and fats.

Unconsciousness — unawareness of and inability to respond to external stimuli and internal needs. (*See also Coma.*)

Uric acid — an end product of purine metabolism. *See Purine.*

Varice, esophageal (adj. variceal) — an enlargement of the branches of a vein connected to the lower esophagus, which are then prone to break open, resulting in severe bleeding.

Vascular spider — dilated capillaries on the skin surface; marked by a spider-like pattern in which red lines radiate from a central dot.

Vasopressor — an agent stimulating muscular tissue contraction in arteries and capillaries.

Ventricle (adj. ventricular) — a small cavity; e.g., one of the lower chambers of the heart.

Venule — a small vein which connects capillaries to a larger vein.

Very heavy drinking — consumption of about 5 drinks per day.

Visuospatial ability — capacity to perform motor skills involving spatial perception, e.g., solve jigsaw puzzles.

Vital sign — a sign of life, e.g., the pulse rate, respiratory rate, body temperature, and blood pressure.

Withdrawal — *see Alcohol withdrawal syndrome.*

Xerostomia — dryness of the mouth.

Appendix A   Selected Resources

NATIONAL INFORMATION CENTERS

American Council on Alcohol Problems (ACAP)
3426 Bridgeland Dr., Bridgeton, MO 63044
1-314-739-5944; fax: 1-314-739-0848
*Comprises religious bodies, and state temperance and fraternal
organizations which work to restrict the availability of alcohol in
the U.S.*

American Council on Alcoholism, Inc.
2522 St. Paul St., Baltimore, MD 21218
1-410-889-0100; fax: 1-410-889-0297
Counseling, referral, and consultation **hot line: 1-800-527-5344**
*Educates the public on alcoholism as a treatable illness. Offers a 12-
hour alcohol education course for drivers. Publishes* ACA NEWS
monthly.

**Assoc. for Medical Education and Research in Substance
Abuse (AMERSA)**
Ctr. for Alcohol and Addiction Studies
Brown University, Box G-BH, Providence, RI 02912
1-401-444-1800
*Serves as a multidisciplinary assoc. of health care professionals.
Provides research materials about substance abuse, emphasizing
medical education.*

Center for Substance Abuse Treatment (CSAT)
Substance Abuse and Mental Health Services Admin. (SAMHSA)
5600 Fishers Lane, Rockville, MD 20857
Publishes Treatment Improvement Protocol (TIP) series, available
from NCADI.
Drug Abuse Information and Treatment Referral **hot line: 1-800-
662-HELP**

Children of Alcoholics Foundation, Inc.
555 Madison Ave., 20th Floor, New York NY 10022
1-800-359-2623 or 212-754-0656
*Offers information, referrals, education, and training on issues
related to addiction*

Natl. Assoc. for Children of Alcoholics (NACoA)
11426 Rockville Pike, Suite 100, Rockville, MD 20852
1-301-468-0985 or 1-888-554-COAS, ext. 2627
Internet: http://www.health.org/nacoa
*Offers support for offspring of alcohol-dependent parents. Publishes
monographs, booklets, and a newsletter to assist professionals in
their patient interventions.*

Natl. Assoc. for Native American Children of Alcoholics
1402 3rd Ave., Suite 1110, Seattle, WA 98101
1-206-467-7686
*Offers substance abuse prevention program, annual conference, and
training for adult children of alcoholics. Provides access to
advocates on local, state, and national levels. Publishes
newsletter.*

Natl. Black Alcoholism Council (NBAC)
285 Genesee St., Utica, NY 13501
1-315-798-8066
*Promotes interaction of African American scholars, alcoholism
professionals, religious leaders, consumers, and human service
providers in solving alcohol-related problems.*

**Natl. Clearinghouse for Alcohol and Drug Information
(NCADI)**
P.O. Box 2345, Rockville, MD 20847-2345
1-800-729-6686; 301-468-2600; TDD: 1-800-487-4889; fax: 1-301-
468-6433
*Provides the public with a wide variety of information on alcohol
misuse and abuse of other drugs.*

Natl. Coalition for Hispanic Health and Human Services
1501 16th St., NW, Washington, DC 20036
1-202-387-5000
*Offers consumer education, outreach training and community-based
model programs, policy analysis, research, advocacy,
development of educational materials on health issues.*

Natl. Council on Alcoholism and Drug Dependence (NCADD)
12 West 21st St., 7th Floor, New York, NY 10010
1-800-622-2255 or 1-212-206-6770; fax: 1-212-645-1690
*Through its many local affiliates, educates Americans about alcohol
misuse and drug addiction . Provides counseling for teenagers
with problems. Publishes educational materials.*

Natl. Institute on Alcohol Abuse and Alcoholism (NIAAA)
Willco Bldg., Suite 409, 6000 Executive Blvd.
Bethesda, MD 20892-7003
1-301-443-3860
Homepage: http://www.niaaa.nih.gov
*Sponsors research on causes, prevention, and treatment of
alcoholism. Publishes* Alcohol Health & Research World *(to order
publications, call* **NCADI** *above).*

Natl. Org. on Fetal Alcohol Syndrome (NOFAS)
1819 H St., NW, Suite 750, Washington, DC 20006
1-202-785-4585 or 1-800-666-6327
*Dedicated to eliminating fetal alcohol syndrome and helping children
and families already affected by alcohol-related birth defects.*

Project Cork Institute
Dartmouth Medical School
7760 Vail Bldg., Hanover, NH 03755
1-603-650-6552
E-mail: cork@Dartmouth.edu
*Promotes health care worker education on substance abuse.
Produces CORK, an on-line database of 25,000 items, available
via Internet and the Dartmouth College Library System.*

Rutgers University Ctr. of Alcoholic Studies
Smithers Hall, Busch Campus, Piscataway, NJ 08855-0969
1-908-445-0787 (voice and fax)
*Conducts research and offers courses on alcohol dependence, its
prevention, and treatment. Provides information to the public and
publishes the* Journal of Studies on Alcohol.

MUTUAL- AND SELF-HELP ANONYMOUS FELLOWSHIPS

Adult Children of Alcoholics (ACOA)
P.O. Box 3216, Torrance, CA 90510
1-310-534-1815
Provides support for family members of alcohol-dependent persons.

Al-Anon Family Group Headquarters
1600 Corporate Landing Parkway, Virginia Beach, VA 23454
1-800-344-2666 (meeting information); 1-800-356-9996 (public outreach); 1-804-563-1600
*Provides information on its local chapters and its affiliated organization, **Alateen**. Both groups are fellowships of persons whose lives have been affected by someone else's drinking.*

Alcoholics Anonymous (A.A.)
World Service Office
P.O. Box 459, Grand Central Station, New York, NY 10164-0371
(corporate address: 475 Riverside Drive, New York, NY 10115)
1-212-870-3400; fax: 1-212-870-3003
Serves as a fellowship of persons who share their experiences so that they may solve their common problems and help others to recover from alcohol dependence (alcoholism). Operates groups for its 12-step program in almost every community.

Rational Recovery Systems (RRS)
P.O. Box 800, Lotus, CA 95651
1-916-621-2667
Serves as a self-help organization, with the philosophy that alcoholics can attain sobriety on their own, without depending on other people or a higher power.

PROFESSIONAL ORGANIZATIONS: PROVIDING ADDICTION TREATMENT INFORMATION AND HELP FOR ADDICTED CLINICIANS

American Dental Assoc. (ADA)
Wellness and Assistance Programs
211 E. Chicago Ave., Chicago, IL 60611
1-312-440-2622, ext. 2622 or 1-800-621-8099, ext. 2622. (*In Canada, dentists should contact the association in their province.*)

American Medical Assoc. (AMA)
Dept. of Mental Health—Physician Health Program
535 Dearborn St., Chicago, IL 60610
1-312-464-5000

American Psychiatric Assoc. (APA)
1400 K St., NW, Washington, DC 20005
1-202-682-6000
Publisher of DSM-IV.

American Society of Addiction Medicine, Inc. (ASAM)
4601 N. Park Ave., Upper Arcade, Suite 101
Chevy Chase, MD 20815-4520
1-301-656-3920; fax: 1-301-656-3815
E-mail: asamoffice@aol.com; home page: http://members.aol.com/asamoffice
Educates physicians on treating persons suffering from alcohol dependence and other addictions. Offers courses and conferences. Publishes the Journal of Addictive Diseases, practice guidelines, a newsletter, and biannual updates for its textbook Principles of Addiction Medicine.

NATIONAL PREVENTION NETWORK: STATE DRUG ABUSE PREVENTION AND TREATMENT OFFICES

Alabama Div. of Substance Abuse Services
200 Interstate Park Dr., Montgomery, AL 36193
1-334-242-3961; fax: 1-334-242-0759

Alaska Council on Prevention of Alcohol and Drug Abuse
3333 Denali St., Suite 201, Anchorage, AK 99503
1-907-258-6021; fax: 1-907-258-6052

American Samoa Alcohol and Drug Programs
Government of American Samoa
Pago Pago, AS 96799
011-684-633-421; fax: 011-684-633-7449

Arizona Drug Abuse Section
Dept. of Health Services
Div. of Behavioral Health Services
2122 E. Highland, Phoenix, AZ 85016
1-602-381-8996; fax: 1-602-553-9143

Arkansas Bureau of Alcohol and Drug Abuse Prevention
5800 W. 10th St., Suite 907, Little Rock, AR 72204
1-501-280-4511; fax: 1-501-280-4519

California Dept. of Alcohol and Drug Programs
1700 K St., 2nd Floor, Sacramento, CA 95814-4037
1-916-327-8617; fax: 1-916-323-0633

Colorado Alcohol and Drug Abuse Div.
Dept. of Human Services
4300 Sherry Creek Dr. S, Denver, CO 80220-1530
1-303-692-2952; fax: 1-303-753-9775

Connecticut Dept. of Mental Health and Addiction Services
410 Capitol Ave., MS14PIT, Hartford, CT 06134
1-860-418-6827; fax: 1-860-418-6792

Delaware Div. of Alcoholism, Drug Abuse, and Mental Health
Office of Prevention
4417 Lancaster Pike, Wilmington, DE 19805
1-302-892-4507; fax: 1-302-633-5114

District of Columbia Office of Prevention and Youth Services
1300 First St., NE, Washington, DC 20018
1-202-727-0092; fax: 1-202-535-2028

Florida HRS Alcohol and Drug Abuse and Mental Health Program
1317 Winewood Blvd., Bldg. B, Rm. 153
Tallahassee, FL 32399-0700
1-904-487-2920, ext 105; fax: 1-904-487-2239

Georgia Substance Abuse Services
Div. of Mental Health, Mental Retardation, and Substance Abuse
2 Peach Tree St., NW, Suite 4-320, Atlanta, GA 30303-3171
1-404-657-2136; fax: 1-404-657-2160

Guam Dept. of Mental Health and Substance Abuse
790 Gov. Carlos G. Camacho Rd., Tamuning, GU 96911
011-671-647-5415; fax: 011-671-649-6948

Hawaii Alcohol and Drug Abuse Div.
1270 Queen Emma St., Rm. 305, Honolulu, HI 96813
1-808-586-4007; fax: 1-808-586-4016

Idaho Bureau of Substance Abuse and Social Services
450 West State St., Boise, ID 83720
1-208-334-5700; fax: 1-208-814-2419

Illinois Dept. of Alcoholism and Substance Abuse
100 W. Randolph St., Suite 5-600, Chicago, IL 60601
1-312-814-6355; fax: 1-312-814-2419

Indiana Div. of Mental Health
402 W. Washington St., W353
Indianapolis, IN 46204-2739
1-317-232-7924; fax: 1-317-233-3472

Iowa Dept. of Public Health
Lucas State Ofc. Bldg.
321 E. 12th St., Des Moines, IA 50319-0075
1-515-281-4404; fax: 1-515-281-4535

Kansas Alcohol and Drug Abuse Services
300 S.W. Oakley, 2nd Floor, Biddle Bldg.
Topeka, KS 66606
1-913-296-3925; fax: 1-913-296-0511-

Kentucky Substance Abuse Div.
1R Health Services Bldg.
275 E. Main St., Frankfort, KY 40621
1-502-564-2880; fax: 1-502-564-3844

Louisiana Div. of Alcohol and Drug Abuse
1201 Capitol Access Rd.
Baton Rouge, LA 70821-3868
1-504-342-9352; fax: 1-504-342-3931

Maine Office of Substance Abuse Prevention and Education Div.
State House Station 159, Augusta, ME 04333
1-207-287-8908; fax: 1-207-287-8910

Maryland Alcohol and Drug Abuse Prevention and Treatment
Services
201 W. Preston St., 4th Floor, Baltimore, MD 21201
1-410-225-6543 (or 6910); fax: 1-410-333-7206

Massachusetts Div. of Substance Abuse Services
150 Tremont St., 6th Floor, Boston, MA 02111
1-617-624-5141; fax: 1-617-624-5185

Michigan Ctr. for Substance Abuse Services
Dept. of Public Health
3423 N. Logan/Martin Luther King Blvd.
Lansing, MI 48909
1-517-335-8843; fax: 1-517-335-8837

Minnesota Chemical Dependency Program Div.
Dept. of Human Services
444 Lafayette Rd., St. Paul, MN 55155-3823
1-612-296-4711; fax: 1-612-297-1862

Mississippi Div. of Alcohol and Drug Abuse
1101 Robert E. Lee Bldg.
239 North Lamar St., Jackson, MI 39201
1-601-359-6216; fax: 1-601-359-6295

Missouri Div. of Alcohol and Drug Abuse
1706 E. Elm St.
P.O. Box 687, Jefferson City, MO 65102
1-314-751-4942; fax: 1-314-751-7814

Montana Addictive and Mental Disorders Div.
Dept. of Public Health and Human Services
1539 11th Ave., Helena, MT 59620
1-406-444-1202; fax: 1-406-444-4435

Nebraska Div. of Alcoholism and Drug Abuse
Dept. of Public Institutions
West Van Dorn and Folsom St.
Lincoln Regional Ctr. Campus, 2nd Floor
Lincoln, NE 68509-4728
1-402-471-2851; fax: 1-402-479-5162

Nevada Bureau of Alcohol and Drug Abuse
Dept. of Human Resources
1830 E. Sahara Ave., Suite 314, Las Vegas, NV 89104
1-702-486-8250; fax: 1-702-486-8253

New Hampshire Office of Alcohol and Drug Abuse Prevention
Manchester, NH 03104-6115
1-603-644-2591; fax: 1-603-622-4043

New Jersey Div. of Alcoholism, Drug Abuse, and Addiction Services
129 E. Hanover St., CN 362, Trenton, NJ 08625
1-609-292-4414; fax: 1-609-292-3816

New Mexico Substance Abuse Bureau
1190 St. Francis Dr., Santa Fe, NM 87503
1-505-827-2601; fax: 1-505-827-0097

New York Office of Alcoholism and Substance Abuse Services
1450 Western Ave., Albany, NY 12203
1-518-485-2123; fax: 1-518-485-2142

North Carolina Alcohol and Drug Abuse Section
325 N. Salisbury St., Suite 531, Raleigh, NC 27611
1-919-733-4555; fax: 1-919-733-9455

North Dakota Div. of Alcoholism and Drug Abuse
1839 East Capitol Ave., Bismarck, ND 58501
1-701-328-9774; fax: 1-701-328-9770

Northern Mariana Islands
Dept. of Public Health Services
P.O. Box 409, Saipan, MP 96950
011-670-323-6560; fax: 011-670-234-8930

Ohio Dept. of Alcohol and Drug Addiction Services
280 N. High St., 12th Floor, Columbus, OH 43215-2357
1-614-466-3445; fax: 1-614-752-8645

Oklahoma Alcohol and Drug Programs
Dept. of Mental Health and Substance Abuse Services
1200 NE 13th, Oklahoma City, OK 73117
1-405-523-3866; fax: 1-405-522-3697

Oregon Dept. of Human Resources
Office of Alcohol and Drug Abuse Programs
500 Summer St., NE, 3rd Floor, Salem, OR 97310-1016
1-503-945-6189; fax: 1-503-378-8467

Pennsylvania Office of Drug and Alcohol Programs
Dept. of Health
Health and Welfare Bldg., Rm. 933
7th and Forester St., Harrisburg, PA 17108
1-717-787-2712; fax: 1-717-787-6285

Puerto Rico Mental Health and Anti-Addiction Services Admin.
P.O. Box 21414, Rio Piedras, PR 00928-1414
1-809-763-3133; fax: 1-809-751-6915

Rhode Island Dept. of Policy Planning and Program Development
Div. of Substance Abuse
25 Howard Ave., Bldg. 57, Cranston, RI 02920
1-401-464-2191; fax: 1-401-464-2089

South Carolina Dept. of Alcohol and Other Drug Abuse Services
3700 Forest Dr., Suite 300, Columbia, SC 29204
1-803-734-9545; fax: 1-803-734-9663

South Dakota Div. of Alcohol and Drug Abuse
Pierre, SD 57501
1-605-773-3123; fax: 1-605-773-5483

Tennessee Bureau of Alcohol and Drug Abuse Services
426 Fifth Ave., N, 3rd Floor, Nashville, TN 37247-4401
1-615-741-1921; fax: 1-615-532-2419

Texas Commission on Alcohol and Drug Abuse
710 Brazos, Suite 403, Austin, TX 78701-2576
1-512-867-8847; fax: 1-512-867-8243

Utah Dept. of Human Services
Div. of Substance Abuse
120 N 200 W, 4th Floor, Salt Lake City, UT 84103
1-801-538-3939; fax: 1-801-438-4696

Vermont Office of Alcohol and Drug Abuse Programs
103 S. Main St., Waterbury, VT 05671-1701
1-802-241-2172; fax: 1-802-241-3095

Virginia Dept. of Mental Health, Mental Retardation, and Substance
Abuse
Office of Substance Abuse Services,12th Floor
P.O. Box 1797, Richmond, VA 23214
1-804-786-1530; fax: 1-804-371-6179

Virgin Islands Div. of Mental Health, Alcohol, and Drug Dependency
#1 Third St., DeCastro Bldg., Sugar Estate, St. Thomas
U.S. Virgin Islands 00802
1-809-774-7700; fax: 1-809-774-4701

Washington Div. of Alcohol and Substance Abuse
Mail Stop: OB-21W
612 Woodland Square Loop SE, Bldg. C, Olympia, WA 98504
1-306-438-8200; fax: 1-360-438-8057

West Virginia Div. of Alcoholism and Drug Abuse
State Capitol Complex, Bldg. 6, Rm. 738, Charleston, WV 25305
1-304-558-2276; fax: 1-304-558-1008

Wisconsin Bureau of Substance Abuse
1 West Wilson St., Rm. 434
P.O. Box 7851, Madison, WI 53707-7851
1-608-266-9485; fax: 1-608-266-1533

Wyoming Alcohol and Drug Abuse Programs
447 Hathaway Bldg., Cheyenne, WY 82002
1-307-777-6493; fax: 1-307-777-5580

Appendix B   Alcohol in Mouthwashes

Dental hygienists, when offering patients mouthwashes to rinse with, should determine preferences: alcohol-containing or nonalcohol mouthwashes. Recovering alcoholics should not use any mouthwash which contains alcohol.

Alcohol in Mouthwashes			
Brand Name	% Alcohol	Brand Name	% Alcohol
Clear Choice®	0	Viadent®	10.0
Rembrandt®	0	Mentadent™ Baking Soda & Peroxide®	12.0
Lavoris®	7.0	Cepacol®	14.0
Plax Mint Sensation®	8.6	Scope Cool Peppermint®	16.6
Plax Original®	8.6	Scope Original Mint®	18.9
Plax SoftMINT®	8.6	Listerine CoolMint®	21.6
Clean Mint Scope (Baking Soda)®	9.8	Listerine Fresh Burst®	21.6

Appendix C   Local Resources Form, To Be Posted

Local Resources for Treatment of Alcohol Misuse and Related Disorders	
Addiction treatment specialists	Name _____ Phone _____ Name _____ Phone _____
Physicians with alcohol-disorder expertise	Name _____ Phone _____ Name _____ Phone _____
State agency	Name Phone
Local A.A. groups	Address _____ Phone _____ Address _____ Phone _____
Community services: <u>residential</u>	Name _____ Phone _____ Contact person _____ Type of facility (circle): adult adolescent
Community services: <u>outpatient</u>	Name _____ Phone _____ Contact person _____ Type of facility (circle): adult adolescent
Community services: <u>evening</u>	Name _____ Phone _____ Contact person _____ Type of facility (circle): adult adolescent
Veterans Affairs services	Name _____ Phone _____ Contact person _____
Other treatment programs	Name _____ Phone _____ Contact person _____ Type of facility (circle): adult adolescent residential outpatient evening Name _____ Phone _____ Contact person _____ Type of facility (circle): adult adolescent residential outpatient evening

Answers to Progress Tests

Progress Test A (Chapters 1 & 2)
1. yeasts
2. 18th
3. personal freedom
4. warning
5. motor vehicle crashes
6. more; more
7. sexual assaults
8. side effects
9. in combination

Progress Test B (Chapters 3 & 4)
1. alcohol dependence
2. live apart
3. disinhibitor
4. extreme sadness
5. peer pressure
6. pure alcohol
7. absorbed; metabolized
8. fatty tissue
9. stops drinking

Progress Test C (Chapters 5 & 6)
1. United States; internationally
2. abuse; dependence
3. tolerance
4. impaired control
5. patient history
6. alcohol misuse
7. parotid gland
8. CAGE
9. GGT

Progress Test D (Chapters 7 & 8)
1. clinical interventions
2. assessments
3. diagnoses
4. ultimately responsible
5. intensive; regular

6. referral
7. when; to whom
8. neurons
9. excitatory; inhibitory

Progress Test E (Chapter 9)
1. intoxicated
2. neuronal
3. cirrhosis
4. vitamin B_1 (thiamine)
5. nerve axons
6. alcoholic dementia
7. abuse potential
8. protracted AWS

Progress Test F (Chapters 10 & 11)
1. lipids
2. >0.25 g/dL
3. nutrient intake
4. mucosa
5. irreversible
6. vasopressor
7. low birth weight
8. elderly
9. aspirin
10. synergistic

Progress Test G (Chapters 12 & 13)
1. >0.15 g/dL
2. quantification
3. controversial
4. monitored
5. opioid
6. Steps; Traditions
7. abstinence violation
8. intrapersonal; interpersonal
9. 8% to 9%

Certificate Request

For the course: <u>Patient Alcohol Abuse:</u>
<u>A Guide for Health Care Professionals</u>

Grade this course on a scale of 1-10 (10 = excellent):   Comment

The material was clearly presented.   _____ _____

The material was logically organized.   _____ _____

The material met the course objectives.   _____ _____

I would recommend this course to others.   _____ _____

I am pleased with HSI's service.   _____ _____

Comments (additional space on the back of this page):

_____

_____

Please tell us what course subjects you would like HSI to develop.

_____

_____

Sign here if we may use your comments in our brochures. _____

For your certificate:

State(s) and license number(s) to be recorded on your certificate _____

_____

Mail my certificate to the name, address, and zip below:

_____ Profession _____

_____

_____

Tear out and send <u>this page</u> with the <u>Scantron answer form</u> to:

HEALTH STUDIES INSTITUTE
P.O.BOX 6808
DEERFIELD BEACH FL
33442-6808

Comments

Index

Reference List for Further Study

1. NIAAA. *The Physicians' Guide to Helping Patients With Alcohol Problems.* U.S. Dept of Health and Human Services, Public Health Service. NIH Publication 95-3769. 1995.
2. NIAAA. *Eighth Special Report to U.S. Congress on Alcohol and Health from the Secretary of Health and Human Services, September 1993.* U.S. Dept of Health and Human Services, Public Health Service. NIH Publication 94-3699. 1994.
3. Rydon P, Redman S. Sanson-Fisher RW, Reid AL. Detection of alcohol-related problems in general practice. *J Stud Alcohol.* 1992;53(3):197-202.
4. Bradley KA. The primary care practitioner's role in the prevention and management of alcohol problems. *Alcohol Health Res World.* 1994;18(2):97-104.
5. Dufour MC. Twenty-five years of alcohol epidemiology. *Alcohol Health Res World.* 1995;19(1):77-16.
6. O'Brien R, Chafetz M. *The Encyclopedia of Alcoholism.* 2nd ed. New York, NY: Facts on File and Greenspring. 1991.
7. Hewitt BG. The creation of the National Institute on Alcohol Abuse and Alcoholism: responding to America's alcohol problem. *Alcohol Health Res World.* 1995;19(1):12-16.
8. Plaut TF. *Alcohol Problems: A report to the nation by the Cooperative Commission on the study of alcoholism.* New York, NY: Oxford University Press. 1967.
9. Meyer RE. The disease called addiction: emerging evidence in a 200-year debate. *Lancet.* January 20, 1996;347:162-166.
10. Marron JT. The Twelve Steps: a pathway to recovery. In: Blondell RD, guest ed. *Substance Abuse: Primary Care.* Philadelphia, Pa: WB Saunders Co. March 1993;20(1):107-119.
11. Gordis E. The National Institute on Alcohol Abuse and Alcoholism: past accomplishments and future goals. *Alcohol Health Res World.* 1995;19(1):5-11.
12. Kirby JM, Maull KI, Fain W. Comparability of alcohol and drug use in injured drivers. *Southern Med J.* 1992;85:800-802.
13. DuPont RL. Laboratory diagnosis. Ch 2 in Section IV: Miller NS, ed. *Principles of Addiction Medicine.* Chevy Chase, MD: ASAM, Inc. 1994.
14. Zobeck TS, Campbell KE, Grant BF, Bertolucci D. *Trends in Alcohol-Related Fatal Traffic Crashes, United States, 1979-1992.* Surveillance Report 30. Rockville, MD: NIAAA. 1994.
15. Wieczorek WF, Welte JW, Abel EL. Alcohol, drugs and murder: a study of convicted homicide offenders. *J Crim Justice.* 1990;18(3):217-227.
16. Welte JW, Abel EL. Homicide: drinking by the victim. *J Stud Alcohol.* 1989;50(3):197-201.
17. Oosterveld WJ. Effect of gravity on positional alcohol nystagmus (PAN). *Aerospace Med.* 1970;41(5):557-560.
18. Morrow D, Von Leirer O, and Yesavage J. The influence of alcohol and aging on radio communication during flight. *Aviat Space Environ Med.* 1990;61(1):12-20.
19. Wintemute GJ, Teret SP, Kraus JF, Wright M. Alcohol and drowning: an analysis of contributing factors and a discussion of criteria for case selection. *Accid Anal Prev.* 1990;22(3):291-296.

20.   Doernberg D, Stinson FS. *U.S. Apparent Consumption of Alcoholic Beverages Based on State Sales, Taxation, or Receipt Data.* Vol. 1. U.S. Alcohol Epidemiologic Data Reference Manual. Washington, DC: U.S. Govt Printing Office. 1985.

21.   Williams GD, Clem DA, Dufour MC. *Apparent Per Capita Alcohol Consumption: National, State, and Regional Trends, 1977-1992.* Surveillance Report 31. Rockville, MD: NIAAA. 1994.

22.   SAMHSA. *National Household Survey on Drug Abuse: Population Estimates 1995.* DHHS Publication (SMA) 96-3095. Rockville, MD: U.S. Dept of Health and Human Services. June 1996.

23.   Mercer PW, Khavari KA. Are women drinking more like men? An empirical examination of the convergence hypothesis. *Alcoholism: Clin Exp Res.* 1990;14(3):461-466.

24.   Blume SB. Women and addictive disorders. Ch 1 in Section XVI: Miller NS, ed. *Principles of Addiction Medicine.* Chevy Chase, MD: ASAM, Inc. 1994.

25.   LaRosa JH. Executive women and health: perceptions and practices. *Am J Public Health.* 1990;80:1450-1454.

26.   Wilsnack SC, Wilsnack RW, Hiller-Sturmhöfel S. How women drink: epidemiology of women's drinking and problem drinking. *Alcohol Health & Res World.* 1994;18(3):173-181.

27.   Crum RM. Epidemiology of addictive disorders. Ch 1 in Section I: Miller NS, ed. *Principles of Addiction Medicine.* Chevy Chase, MD: ASAM, Inc. 1994.

28.   NIAAA. College students and drinking. *Alcohol Alert.* July 1995;29:1-4.

29.   Caetano R. Alcohol use among Hispanic groups in the United States. *Am J Drug Alcohol Abuse.* 1988;14(3):293-308.

30.   Suddendorf RF. Research on alcohol metabolism among Asians and its implications for understanding causes of alcoholism. *Public Health Rep.* 1989;104(6):615-620.

31.   Chi I, Lubben JE, Kitano HHL. Differences in drinking behavior among three Asian-American groups. *J Stud on Alcohol.* 1989;50(1):15-23.

32.   Champion HR, Copes WS, Sacco WJ, et al. The major trauma care outcome study: establishing national norms for trauma care. *J of Trauma.* 1990;30:1356-1365.

33.   Soderstrom CA. Detecting alcohol-related problems in trauma center patients. *Alcohol Health Res World.* 1994;18(2):127-130.

34.   SAMHSA. *Preliminary Estimates from the Drug Abuse Warning Network: 1995 drug-related emergency department episodes.* Advance Report 17. DHHS Publication (SMA) 96-3106. Rockville, MD: U.S. Dept of Health and Human Services. August 1996.

35.   SAMHSA. *Annual Medical Examiner Data, 1993.* Statistical Series I, No. 13-B. DHHS Publication (SMA) 95-3019. Rockville MD: U.S. Dept of Health and Human Services. 1995.

36.   Merikangas KR. The genetic epidemiology of alcoholism. *Psychol Med.* 1990;20:11-22.

37.   Cloninger CR. Neurogenetic adaptive mechanisms in alcoholism. *Science.* 1987;236:410-416.

38.   Anthenelli RM, Schuckit MA. Genetics. Ch 4 in: Lowinson JH, Ruiz P, Millman RB, eds. *Substance Abuse: A Comprehensive Textbook.* 2nd ed. Baltimore, MD: Williams & Wilkins. 1992.

39.   Ball SA, Kosten TA. Diagnostic classification systems. Ch 6 in Section IV: Miller NS, ed. *Principles of Addiction Medicine.* Chevy Chase, MD: ASAM, Inc. 1994.

40.   Cadoret RJ. Genetics of alcoholism. Pages 39-78 in: Collins RL, Leonard KE, Searles JS, eds. *Alcohol and the Family: Research and Clinical Perspectives.* New York, NY: Guilford Press. 1990.

41.   McGue M, Pickens RW, Svikis DS. Sex and age effects on the inheritance of alcohol problems: A twin study. *J Abnorm Psychol.* 1992;101(1):3-17.

42.   Davis PA, Gibbs FA, Favis H, et al. The effects of alcohol upon the electroencephalogram. *J Stud Alcohol.* 1941;1:626-637.

43.   Ehlers CL, Schuckit MA. EEG fast frequency activity in sons of alcoholics. *Biol Psychiatry.* 1990;27(6):631-641.

44. Rausch JL, Monteiro MG, Schuckit MA. Platelet serotonin uptake in men with family histories of alcoholism. *Neuropsychopharmacology.* 1992;4(2):83-86.

45. Schuckit MA, Gold E, Risch C. Plasma cortisol levels following ethanol in sons of alcoholics and controls. *Arch Gen Psychiatry.* 1987;44(11):942-945.

46. Schuckit MA, Gold E, Risch C. Serum prolactin levels in sons of alcoholics and control subjects. *Arch J Psychiatry.* 1987;144(7):854-859.

47. Finn PR, Pihl RO. Risk for alcoholism: A comparison between two different groups of sons of alcoholics on cardiovascular reactivity and sensitivity to alcohol. *Alcoholism: Clin Exp Res.* 1988;12(6):742-747.

48. Blum K, Noble EP, Sheridan PJ, et al. Allelic association of human dopamine D2 receptor gene in alcoholism. *JAMA.* 1990;263(15):2055-2060.

49. Marlatt GA. Alcohol, the magic elixir: Stress, expectancy, and the transformation of emotional states. Pages 302-322 in: Gottheil E, Druly KA et al., eds. *Stress and Addiction.* New York, NY: Brunner/Mazel. 1987.

50. Steele CM, Josephs RA. Alcohol myopia: Its prized and dangerous effects. *Am Psychol.* 1990;45(8):921-933.

51. Newlin DB, Thomson JB. Alcohol challenge with sons of alcoholics: A critical review and analysis. *Psychol Bulletin.* 1990;108(3):383-402.

52. Sher KJ. Stress response dampening. Pages 227-271 in: Blane HT, Leonard KE, eds. *Psychological Theories of Drinking and Alcoholism.* New York, NY: Guilford Press. 1987.

53. Leigh BC. The relationship of sex-related alcohol expectancies to alcohol consumption and sexual behavior. *Br J Addict.* 1990;85(7):919-928.

54. Norris J. Alcohol and female sexuality. *Alcohol Health Res World.* 1994;18(3):197-201.

55. Harburg E, Davis DR, Caplan R. Parent and offspring alcohol use: Imitative and aversive transmission. *J Stud Alcohol.* 1982;43(5):497-516.

56. Barnes GM, Garrell MP, Cairns A. Parental socialization factors and adolescent drinking behaviors. *J Marriage Family.* 1986;48(1):27-36.

57. Kandel DB, Andrews K. Processes of adolescent socialization by parents and peers. *Int J Addict.* 1987;22(4):319-342.

58. Ringwalt CL, Palmer JH. Differences between white and black youth who drink heavily. *Addict Behav.* 1990;15:455-460.

59. Holmes SJ, Robins LNN. The influence of childhood disciplinary experiences on the development of alcoholism and depression. *J Child Psychol Psychiatry.* 1987;28(3):399-415.

60. Morgan M, Grube JW. Closeness and peer group influence. *Br J Soc Psychol.* 1991;30:159-161.

61. Alexander F, Duff RW. Social interaction and alcohol use in retirement communities. *Gerontologist.* 1988;28:632-638.

62. Wallach L, Grube JW, Madden PA, et al. Portrayals of alcohol on prime-time television. *J Stud Alcohol.* 1990;51(5):428-437.

63. Goodwin DW. *Alcoholism: The Facts.* 2nd ed. Oxford, Great Britain: Oxford University Press. 1994.

64. Woolf DS. CNS depressants: alcohol. Ch 2 in Bennett EG, Woolf DS, eds. *Substance Abuse: Pharmacologic, Developmental and Clinical Perspectives.* 2nd ed. Albany, NY: Delmar Publishers, Inc. 1991.

65 Berberoglu H. *An Introduction to Alcoholic Beverages.* Toronto, Ontario: Ryerson Polytechnical Institute. 1987.

66. Becker CE, Roe RL, Scott RA. *Alcohol as a Drug: A curriculum on pharmacology, neurology and toxicology.* Huntington, NY: Robert E. Krieger Publishing Co. 1979.

67. Schuckit MA. Alcoholism and drug dependency. Ch 390 in: Isselbacher KJ, Braunwald E, Wilson JD, et al, eds. *Harrison's Principles of Internal Medicine.* 13th ed. New York, NY: McGraw-Hill; 1994.

68. Goldstein DB. Pharmacokinetics of alcohol. Ch 2 in: Mendelson JH, Mello NK, eds. *Medical Diagnosis and Treatment of Alcoholism.* New York, NY: McGraw-Hill. 1992.

69. Woodward JJ. Alcohol. Ch 2 in Section II: Miller NS, ed. *Principles of Addiction Medicine.* Chevy Chase, MD: ASAM, Inc. 1994.

70. Lieber CS. Medical disorders of alcoholism. *NEJM.* October 19, 1995;333(16):1058-1065.

71. Deal, SR, Gavaler JS. Are women more susceptible than men to alcohol-induced cirrhosis? *Alcohol Health Res World.* 1994;18(3)189-191.

72. Lowe G. Alcohol and alcoholism. Ch 4 in: Sanger DJ, Blackman DE, ed. *Aspects of Psychopharmacology.* Psychology in Progress Series. London, England: Methuen & Co. 1984.

73. Charness ME. Molecular mechanisms of ethanol intoxication, tolerance, and physical dependence. Chapter 5 in: Mendelson JH, Mello NK, eds. *Medical Diagnosis and Treatment of Alcoholism.* New York, NY: McGraw-Hill. 1992.

74. American Psychiatric Association. *Diagnostic and Statistical Manual of Mental Disorders, DSM-IV.* 4th ed. Washington, DC: American Psychiatric Association. 1994.

75. Victor M. The effects of alcohol on the nervous system. Ch 6 in: Mendelson JH, Mello NK, eds. *Medical Diagnosis and Treatment of Alcoholism.* New York, NY: McGraw-Hill. 1992.

76. WHO. *The ICD-10 Classification of Mental and Behavioural Disorders: Clinical descriptions and diagnostic guidelines.* 10th rev. Geneva: World Health Organization. 1992.

77. NIAAA. Diagnostic criteria for alcohol abuse and dependence. *Alcohol Alert.* October 1995;30:1-6.

78. Grant BF, Harford TC, Dawson DA, et al. Prevalence of DSM-IV alcohol abuse and dependence. *Alcohol Health Res World.* 1994;18(3):243-248.

79. Brostoff WS. Clinical diagnosis. Ch 1 in Section IV: Miller NS, ed. *Principles of Addiction Medicine.* Chevy Chase, MD: ASAM, Inc. 1994.

80. NIAAA. Alcohol and tolerance. *Alcohol Alert.* April 1995;28(PH356):1-4.

81. Linnoila M, Colburn TR, Petersen RC. On the research front: the NIAAA intramural research program. *Alcohol Health Res World.* 1995;19(1):60-70.

82. McCusker CG, Brown K. Alcohol-predictive cues enhance tolerance to and precipitate "craving" for alcohol in social drinkers. *J Stud Alcohol.* 1990;51(6):494-499.

83. Sdao-Jarvie K, Vogel-Sprott M. Response expectancies affect the acquisition and display of behavioral tolerance to alcohol. *Alcohol.* 1991;8(6):491-498.

84. Vogel-Sprott M, Rawana E, Webster R. Mental rehearsal of a task under ethanol facilitates tolerance. *Pharmacol Biochem Behav.* 1984;21(3):329-331.

85. Babor TF. Diagnosis of alcohol abuse and dependence. Ch 1 in: Mendelson JH, Mello NK, eds. *Medical Diagnosis and Treatment of Alcoholism.* New York, NY: McGraw-Hill. 1992.

86. Bissell L. Diagnosis and recognition. In: Bitlow SE, Peyser, HS, eds. *Alcoholism: A Practical Treatment Guide.* New York, NY: Grune & Stratton. 1980.

87. Iber FL. *Alcohol and Drug Abuse as Encountered in Office Practice.* Boca Raton, FL: CRC Press, Inc. 1991.

88. Buchsbaum DG. Quick, effective screening for alcohol abuse. *Patient Care.* July 15, 1995: 56-69.

89. Council on Dental Practice. *ADA Oral Health Care Guidelines: Chemically Dependent Patients.* Chicago, IL: American Dental Association. May 1993.

90. O'Connor PG. The general internist. *Alcohol Health Res World.* 1994;18(2):110-116.

91. Maly RC. Early recognition of chemical dependence. In: Blondell RD, guest ed. *Substance Abuse: Primary Care.* Philadelphia, Pa: WB Saunders Co. March 1993;20(1):33-50.

92. Comerci GD. Office assessment and brief intervention with the addicted adolescent. Ch 2 in Section XVII: Miller NS, ed. *Principles of Addiction Medicine.* Chevy Chase, MD: ASAM, Inc. 1994.

93. Fleming MF. Screening and brief intervention for alcohol disorders. *J Fam Pract.* 1993;37(3):231-234.

94. Nilssen O, Hunter C. Screening patients for alcohol problems in primary health care settings. *Alcohol Health Res World.* 1994;18(2):136-139.

95. Babor TF, Grant M. From clinical research to secondary prevention: international collaboration in the development of the Alcohol Use Disorders Identification Test (AUDIT). *Alcohol Health Res World.* 1989;13(4):371-374.

96. Drucker F. Mandatory reporting of loss of consciousness or confusion due to alcohol. *JAMA.* June 21, 1995; 273(23):1833 (letter).

97. Kitchens J. Mandatory reporting of loss of consciousness or confusion due to alcohol. *JAMA.* June 21, 1995; 273(23):1833 (reply to letter).

98. Russell M. New assessment tools for risk drinking during pregnancy: T-ACE, TWEAK, and others. *Alcohol Health Res World.* 1994;18(1):55-61.

99. Salaspuro M. Biological state markers of alcohol abuse. *Alcohol Health Res World.* 1994;18(2):131-135.

100. Allen JP, Litten RZ. Biochemical and psychometric tests. Ch 3 in Section IV: Miller NS, ed. *Principles of Addiction Medicine.* Chevy Chase, MD: ASAM, Inc. 1994.

101. Dubowski KM. *The Technology of Breath-Alcohol Analysis.* DHHS Publication (ADM) 92-1728. Rockville, MD: NIAAA. 1992.

102. Seppä K, Laippala P, Saarni M. Macrocytosis as a consequence of alcohol abuse among patients in general practice. *Alcoholism: Clin Exp Res.* 1991;15(5):871-876.

103. Steindler EM. Addiction terminology. Ch 2 in Section I: Miller NS, ed. *Principles of Addiction Medicine.* Chevy Chase, MD: ASAM, Inc. 1994.

104. Graham AW. Brief intervention. Ch 7 in Section IV: Miller NS, ed. *Principles of Addiction Medicine.* Chevy Chase, MD: ASAM, Inc. 1994

105. Benzer DG, Winslow TF. Formal interventions. Ch 8 in Section IV: Miller NS, ed. *Principles of Addiction Medicine.* Chevy Chase, MD: ASAM, Inc. 1994.

106. Gastfriend DR, Najavits LM, Reif S. Assessment instruments. Ch 4 in Section IV: Miller NS, ed. *Principles of Addiction Medicine.* Chevy Chase, MD: ASAM, Inc. 1994.

107. Lewis DC. Medical and behavioral management of alcohol problems in general medical practice. Ch 13 in: Mendelson JH, Mello NK, eds. *Medical Diagnosis and Treatment of Alcoholism.* New York, NY: McGraw-Hill. 1992.

108. Botelho RJ, Novak S. Dealing with substance misuse, abuse, and dependency. In: Blondell RD, guest ed. *Substance Abuse: Primary Care.* Philadelphia, Pa: WB Saunders Co. March 1993;20(1):51-70.

109. U.S. Dept of Agriculture. *Dietary Guidelines, Nutrition and Your Health.* 3rd ed. Publication 1990-273-930. Washington, DC: U.S. Govt Printing Office. 1990.

110 Sanchez-Craig M, Lei H. Disadvantages of imposing the goal of abstinence on problem drinkers: an empirical study. *Br J Addict.* 1986;81(4):505-512.

111. Barry KL, Fleming MF. The family physician. *Alcohol Health Res World.* 1994;18(2):105-109.

112. McCaul ME, Furst J. Alcoholism treatment in the United States. *Alcohol Health Res World.* 1994;18(4):253-260.

113. Lopez F. *Confidentiality of Patient Records for Alcohol and Other Drug Treatment.* Tech. Assistance Publication Series 13. DHHS Publication (SMA) 95-3018. SAMHSA. 1994

114. Holbrook JM. The autonomic and central nervous systems. Ch 1 in Bennett EG, Woolf DS, eds. *Substance Abuse: Pharmacologic, Developmental and Clinical Perspectives.* 2nd ed. Albany, NY: Delmar Publishers, Inc. 1991.

115. Society for Neuroscience. *Brain Facts: A primer on the brain and nervous system.* Washington, DC: Society for Neuroscience. 1990.

116. Hiller-Sturmhöfel S. Signal transmission among nerve cells. *Alcohol Health Res World.* 1995;19(2):128.

117. Geller A. Neurological effects. Ch 6 in Section V: Miller NS, ed. *Principles of Addiction Medicine.* Chevy Chase, MD: ASAM, Inc. 1994.

118. Butterworth RG. The role of liver disease in alcohol-induced cognitive defects. *Alcohol Health Res World.* 1995;19(2):122-129.

119. Langlais PJ. Alcohol-related thiamine deficiency: impact on cognitive and memory functioning. *Alcohol Health Res World.* 1995;19(2):113-121.

120. Cutting J. The relationship between Korsakoff's syndrome and "alcoholic dementia." *Br J Psychiatry.* 1978;132:240-251.

121. Wartenberg AA. Medical syndromes associated with specific drugs. Ch 2 in Section V: Miller NS, ed. *Principles of Addiction Medicine.* Chevy Chase, MD: ASAM, Inc. 1994.

122. Anton RF. Medications for treating alcoholism. *Alcohol Health Res World.* 1994;18(4):265-271.

123. Gastfriend DR. Pharmacologic treatment of dual diagnosis. Ch 6 in Section VI: Miller NS, ed. *Principles of Addiction Medicine.* Chevy Chase, MD: ASAM, Inc. 1994.

124. Miller NS. Psychiatric comorbidity: occurrence and treatment. *Alcohol Health Res World.* 1994;18(4):261-264.

125. Schuckit M, Irwin M, Brown S. The history of anxiety symptoms among 171 primary alcoholics. *J Stud Alcohol.* 1990;51:34-41.

126. Schuckit MA. *Drug and Alcohol Abuse: A clinical guide to diagnosis and treatment.* New York, NY: Plenum Publishing Corp. 1989.

127. ASAM. Management of acute episodes. Ch 1 in Section XI: Miller NS, ed. *Principles of Addiction Medicine.* Chevy Chase, MD: ASAM, Inc. 1994.

128. Webb RM, Schneider DM. Ophthalmology. Ch 7 in Section VII: Miller NS, ed. *Principles of Addiction Medicine.* Chevy Chase, MD: ASAM, Inc. 1994.

129. Feinman L, Lieber CS. Nutrition. Ch 8 in Section V: Miller NS, ed. *Principles of Addiction Medicine.* Chevy Chase, MD: ASAM, Inc. 1994.

130. Colditz GA, Giovannucci E, Rimm EB, et al. Alcohol intake in relation to diet and obesity in women and men. *Am J Clin Nutr.* 1991;54(1):49-55.

131. U.S. Dept of Health and Human Services. *The Surgeon General's Report on Nutrition and Health.* DHHS Publication PHS88-50210. Washington, DC: U.S. Govt Printing Office. 1988.

132. NIAAA. Alcohol and nutrition. *Alcohol Alert.* Publication PH346. October 1993;22:1-4.

133. Korsten MA, Lieber CS. Organ pathology. Ch 5 in Section V: Miller NS, ed. *Principles of Addiction Medicine.* Chevy Chase, MD: ASAM, Inc. 1994.

134. Sherlock S, Dooley J. *Diseases of the Liver and Biliary System.* 9th ed. Oxford, England: Blackwell Scientific Publications. 1993.

135. Singh M. Ethanol and the pancreas: current status. *Gastroenterology.* 1990;98:1051-1062.

136. Korsten MA. Alcoholism and pancreatitis: does nutrition play a role? *Alcohol Health Res World.* 1989;13:232-237.

137. Korsten MA, Lieber CS. The gastrointestinal effects of alcohol. Ch 8 in: Mendelson JH, Mello NK, eds. *Medical Diagnosis and Treatment of Alcoholism.* New York, NY: McGraw-Hill. 1992.

138. Chang DJ. Of all the ginned joints. *Patient Care.* March 15, 1996;30(5):182-184.

139. NIAAA. Alcohol and hormones. *Alcohol Alert.* October 1994;26(PH352):1-4.

140. McKinley CR, Tremblay RE. Genitourinary disorders. Ch 8 in Section VII: Miller NS, ed. *Principles of Addiction Medicine.* Chevy Chase, MD: ASAM, Inc. 1994.

141. Thorp JM Jr, with Hiller-Sturmhöfel S. The obstetrician/gynecologist. *Alcohol Health Res World.* 1994;18(2):117-120.

142. Jones TB, Smith RS, Martier S, et al. Alcohol and drug use in pregnancy: effects on the offspring. Ch 5 in Section XVI: Miller NS, ed. *Principles of Addiction Medicine.* Chevy Chase, MD: ASAM, Inc. 1994.

143. Miller LJ. Detoxification of the addicted women in pregnancy. Ch 3 in Section XVI: Miller NS, ed. *Principles of Addiction Medicine.* Chevy Chase, MD: ASAM, Inc. 1994.

144. NIAAA. Alcohol-medication interactions. *Alcohol Alert.* January 1995;27(PH355):1-4.

145   Egbert AM. The older alcoholic: recognizing the subtle clinical clues. *Geriatrics.* 1993;48(7):63-69.

146.   Guram MS, Howden CW, Holt S. Alcohol and drug interactions. *Practical Gastroenterology.* 1992;16(8):47-54.

147.   Jatlow P, Ellsworth JD, Bradberry CW, et al. Cocaethylene: a neuropharmacologically active metabolite associated with concurrent cocaine-ethylene ingestion. *Life Sciences.* 1991;48:1787-1794.

148.   Benzer DG. Management of alcohol intoxication and withdrawal. Ch 3 in Section XI: Miller NS, ed. *Principles of Addiction Medicine.* Chevy Chase, MD: ASAM, Inc. 1994.

149.   SAMHSA. *Pregnant, Substance-Using Women.* Treatment Improvement Protocol (TIP) Series 2. DHHS Publication (SMA)93-1998. Center for Substance Abuse Treatment. 1993.

150.   Benzer DG. Quantification of the alcohol withdrawal syndrome in 487 alcoholic patients. *J Subst Abuse Treat.* 1990;7:117-123.

151.   Sullivan JT, Sykora K, Schneiderman J, et al. *Br J Addict. 1989;84:1353-1357.*

152.   Kurtzweill P. Medications can aid recovery from alcoholism. *FDA Consumer.* May 1996;30(4):22-25.

153.   Kasser C. The role of phenytoin in the management of alcohol withdrawal syndrome. ASAM Clinical Practice Guide. Ch 10 in Section XI: Miller NS, ed. *Principles of Addiction Medicine.* Chevy Chase, MD: ASAM, Inc. 1994.

154.   Lechtenberg R, Worner TM. Prospective study of seizure risk management of alcoholics during in-patient detoxification. *International Symposium on Alcohol and Seizures.* Washington, D.C. 1988.

155.   Malcolm RJ, Ballenger JC, Sturgis E, Anton RF. A double-blind controlled trial comparing carbamazepine to oxazepam treatment of alcohol withdrawal. *Am J Psychiatry.* 1989;146:617-621.

156.   Chick J, Gough K, Falkowski W, et al. Disulfiram treatment of alcoholism. *Br J Psychiatry.* 1992;161:84-89.

157.   Philips M. Depot disulfiram: pharmacokinetics and clinical effects during 28 days following a single subcutaneous dose. In: Naranjo CA, Sellers EM, eds. *Novel Pharmacological Interventions for Alcoholism.* New York: Springer-Verlag. 1992:273-276.

158.   Peachey JE, Annis HM, Bornstein ER, et al. Calcium carbimide in alcoholism treatment. Part 1: A placebo-controlled, double-blind clinical trial of short-term efficacy. *Br J Addict.* 1989;84(4):877-887.

159.   Keung WM, Vallee BI. Daidzin and daidzein suppress free-choice ethanol intake by Syrian golden hamsters. *Proc Natl Acad Sci, USA.* 1993:90:10008-10012.

160.   Whitworth AB, Fischer F, Lesch OM, et al. Comparison of acamprosate and placebo in long-term treatment of alcohol dependence. *Lancet.* May 25, 1996;347(9013):1438-1442.

161.   Volpicelli JR, Clay KL, Watson NT, Volpicelli LA. Naltrexone and the treatment of alcohol dependence. *Alcohol Health Res World.* 1994;18(4):272-278.

162.   Volpicelli JR, Alterman AI, Hayashida M, O'Brien CP. Naltrexone in the treatment of alcohol dependence. *Arch Gen Psychiatry.* 1992;49(11):876-880.

163.   O'Malley SS, Jaffe AJ, Chang G, et al. Naltrexone and coping skills therapy for alcohol dependence: a controlled study. *Arch Gen Psychiatry.* 1992;49(11):881-887.

164.   Swift RM, Whelihan W, Kuznetsov O, et al. Naltrexone-induced alterations in human ethanol intoxication. *Am J Psychiatry.* October 1994;151(10):1463-1467.

165.   Mattson ME. Patient-treatment matching: rationale and results. *Alcohol Health Res World.* 1994;18(4):287-295.

166.   Ludwig AM. *The Nature of Craving and How to Control It.* New York, NY: Oxford University Press. 1988.

167.   Tonigan JS, Hiller-Sturmhöfel S. Alcoholics Anonymous: who benefits? *Alcohol Health Res World.* 1994;18(4):308-309..

168.   Schulz JE. Twelve step programs. Ch 2 in Section XIV: Miller NS, ed. *Principles of Addiction Medicine*. Chevy Chase, MD: ASAM, Inc. 1994.

169.   Schulz JE, Chappel J. The physician's role in twelve-step programs. Ch 1 in Section XIV: Miller NS, ed. *Principles of Addiction Medicine*. Chevy Chase, MD: ASAM, Inc. 1994.

170.   DuPont RL, Shiraki S. Recent research in twelve step programs. Ch 5 in Section XIV: Miller NS, ed. *Principles of Addiction Medicine*. Chevy Chase, MD: ASAM, Inc. 1994.

171.   Woititz J. *Adult Children of Alcoholics*. Pompano Beach, FL: Health Communications, Inc. 1981.

172.   Kadden RM. Cognitive-behavioral approaches to alcoholism treatment. *Alcohol Health Res World*. 1994;18(4):279-286.

173.   Marlatt GA. Relapse prevention: theoretical rationale and overview of the model. Pages 3-32 in: Marlatt GA, Gordon JR, eds. *Relapse Prevention*. New York, NY: Guilford Press. 1985.

174.   Marlatt GA, Gordon JR, eds. *Relapse Prevention*. New York, NY: Guilford Press. 1985.

175.   Monti PM, Abrams DB, Kadden RM, et al. *Treating Alcohol Dependence: A coping skills training guide*. New York, NY: Guilford Press. 1989.

176.   Galanter M. Network therapy: a model for office practice. Ch 3 in Section XIII: Miller NS, ed. *Principles of Addiction Medicine*. Chevy Chase, MD: ASAM, Inc. 1994.

177.   Wells-Parker E. Mandated treatment: lessons from research with drinking and driving offenders. *Alcohol Health Res World*. 1994;18(4):302-306.